OVERUSE INJURIES:

Their Prevention and Treatment

By David Enos

Dedicated to:

This book is affectionately dedicated to my wife Marcia, who has given so much emotional support through the writing of it and has been my <u>best friend</u> through all of it; to my parents, Gerry and Nanci, for their love and support; to Dr. Donald Jones for his help, advice, and constant humanitarianism; to Kelly Coleman for her legal advice and friendship; to Jim Britt for his fantastic pictures and friendship; my teachers, Frank Sumares and Gil Cline, for their friendship, their belief in my abilities and their dedication to education; and finally, to all the people I've talked to along the way who have given me advice, tips, experience, or most of all, **hope**-this book is for you.

DISCLAIMER

The research and personal experiences of the author form the sole basis for the information and suggestions presented in this book. The author strongly recommends that the reader consult his/her physician (or any other qualified health care professional) prior to incorporating any of the material contained in this book into a personal health regimen. The author assumes no responsibility whatsoever for any adverse reactions or consequences occasioned by the reader's use of any of the information and/or suggestions contained herein.

FOREWORD

By Donald E. Jones, DC, ND, PT, BA, BS, MS, Ph.D., BCDp.NT(103147) Doctor / Author / Laureate

This is an important book - important to laymen, and important to physicians and scientists interested in the health of people.

David Enos deserves much credit for having marshaled the arguments that indicate that most human beings have been receiving amounts of ascorbic acid less than those required to put them in the best of health. It is his contention, and it is supported by much evidence, that most people in the world have conditions involving a deficient intake of varied healthful substances.

For many millions of years now, until recently, man has obtained ample amounts of all nutrients from the food consumed. Unfortunately, our soil depletion of nutrients has diminished to an all time low, due to modern farming practices and plowing. In fact, a Congressional Report in 1936 presented to congress showed that every 10 years our soils reduce by 50%. The representative was worried about future generations to come.

Congress never acted, however, and a company called ADM (Archer-Daniels-Midland), started selling 100lb. sacks of "PNP", sold all over the world, just to make everything grow with good appearance. We are not supposed to know the difference. PNP (or Phosphorus, Nitrogen & Potassium) lacks most of the trace minerals needed for good abundant health. We have been 'scammed'. In that light, we must all consume 'added' nutrients for the sake of our personal health as well as future generations.

David Enos has done a fine job of describing what is needed in his publication. Every year the population of this world increases; however, the nutrients decrease. It is very likely that we as human beings in this present day are receiving less than 2% of the nutrients found naturally in past generations. David has summarized this information and evidence, telling it like it is for any person suffering. Anyone reading this can expect great improvement, when followed.

As a Board Certified Diplomat in Nutritional Therapy, and having reviewed David's writings, I feel comfortable in recommending this book.

TABLE OF CONTENTS

WHY SHOULD YOU OWN THIS BOOK?

1) **I've been there**. I'm a professional musician who suffered from tendonitis, bone spurs, and carpal tunnel syndrome for eight years and made a complete and total recovery. I no longer suffer from overuse injuries. I understand what you're going through and believe many of the things in this book will work for you, not only because they worked for me but for many of my friends as well.

2) **My experiences are varied**. I saw a variety of health care professionals during the eight years I suffered from overuse injuries: doctors, nutritionists, chiropractors, acupuncturists, myotherapists, etc. I spent numerous hours reading about overuse injuries, not only in books and magazines but looking up studies pertaining to overuse injuries in publications such as the New England Journal of Medicine. These varied experiences have kept me from taking one line of thought when approaching overuse problems. Every health care approach has something to offer. I've listed the best methods from each approach.

3) **This book is written in easy-to-understand laymen's terms**. I don't have a health care degree but I have included treatments that really work. These treatments have been helpful to myself as well as others.

In short, if you have overuse injuries or want to prevent overuse injuries, this book is for you. I am confident in these treatments because I know they work. They literally saved my career. I wish you the best of luck and health in your quest for a pain-free life. Your body has the capability of healing itself if you give it the proper tools - believe it. This worked for me and I believe it can work for you.

INTRODUCTION

It's a widely accepted thought among health care professionals (as well as musicians) that overuse injuries are permanent once you've gotten them. There was a time when I believed this. I had spent eight years and a lot of money visiting doctors, neurologists, chiropractors, acupuncturists, etc. I had seen virtually everyone that had any relevance to my problems and nothing seemed to help. Extended practicing and overworking for six months solid caused the onset of tendonitis, bone spurs, and carpal tunnel syndrome; but now that I had these maladies, what was I to do?

My situation appeared hopeless. It came down to three choices: surgery, learn to play the bass right-handed after 16 years (I'm left - handed), or find a new career. I began to seriously consider surgery when I came across several experts in the health care industry that saved my career. Each discipline offered different treatments that proved beneficial. Slowly, over a period of about a year, my suffering began to diminish. I am currently living a life without the pain from these injuries. What follows are things I learned from the process.

The state of your body is not constant. It varies from hour to hour and day to day. How you feel at a given moment can be a result of temperature (internal or environmental), how rested or stressed you are, diet, how much you've overworked your body prior to that moment, and other factors.

Nutrition, **muscle conditioning**, **playing habits**, **rest**, and **psychological state** are the five main areas that affect an overuse injury. In addition to helping overuse injuries, other benefits of addressing these areas may include better physical health, weight loss, and/or a more relaxed state of mind. We will expand on each of these areas in subsequent chapters.

Making the required changes in your lifestyle requires discipline. You may think these changes are limiting. As a point of fact, overuse injuries are more limiting than the self-discipline required for preventing or healing them. All five prior-mentioned areas need to be addressed when dealing with overuse injuries. It is not enough to deal solely with nutrition and rest while neglecting the other three areas.

It takes time to heal so be patient. Don't expect miracles overnight. If you currently have an overuse injury you know how long it took you to acquire it. It may take some time to reverse the damage. Remember that your body is always trying to repair itself. Under the right conditions it can take as little as three days for your body to heal from some injuries.

Learn moderation. You wouldn't rub a cut on your skin that's been stitched because it would slow down the healing process. Yet this is essentially what you do to your muscles every time you practice/work long hours with an overuse injury. Give your body a chance to heal and rebuild. This might mean taking a vacation from your job, a break from your instrument, or limiting your time at work or practice.

Learn moderation in all five areas of your lifestyle. Don't binge on junk food, get adequate sleep, don't over-exercise, keep your emotions in check, and don't spend excessive hours practicing/working. Find peace in moderation and make these changes now.

Continue trying the various remedies presented until you find combinations that work for you. It is extremely encouraging to find a remedy that helps. It helps you maintain a positive attitude and gives you hope about curing your injury.

You must supply your body with the tools it needs for repair. Nutrition and exercise apply here. Drugs may relieve pain quickly but are temporary only. They do little for the underlying cause of the pain. The concept is healing your body naturally. Natural healing is slow but it is permanent. Your nutrient and oxygen levels affect how quickly your body heals. Correct nutrition and aerobic exercise supply nutrients and oxygen necessary for regeneration.

Keep a daily journal to see if there is a correlation between how you feel and the part of your lifestyle you've changed. This is an extremely helpful part of the process so don't neglect it. It is impossible to remember what you've had to eat over the course of a week. Keeping a journal will help show correlations between dietary changes, exercise changes, and so on. Be sure to include the date, time, emotional state you were in, what you were doing, your diet, the time you woke/went to sleep, etc.

Most people go through withdrawal symptoms when they alter their habits and lifestyle. These symptoms may manifest in various ways. Some examples may include pain moving around to different areas (re-appearing in areas that seemed to be healed) or moving to the same place on the opposite side of your body. Remember that changes in your lifestyle result in changes in your body. Your cells regenerate, your chemical and PH balances change, and it is typical to feel like you are regressing a little when in reality you are improving. Don't get discouraged.

Finally, **We are all genetically different.** What works for me may not work for you and vice versa. It wasn't unusual to talk to people who swore by DMSO when it had no effect on me. I've presented many options to pick and choose from until you find the combination of treatments that help you the most. You know your body better than anyone else. Listen to it.

CHAPTER 1: NUTRITION

SUPPLEMENTS

Supplements are an important part of the healing process. A typical American diet is comprised of food stripped of vitamins, minerals, enzymes and hormones. These vitamins, minerals, enzymes and hormones are the tools your body needs for repair. Not surprisingly, many supplements that promote tissue repair (like vitamins C or E) have anti-aging properties as well. You may find your wrinkles are less noticeable when you take vitamin E, for example. The most important supplements for tissue repair are those known as anti-oxidants. These supplements increase oxygen in muscle tissues, thereby slowing down oxidation.

What does oxidation have to do with overuse injuries? To illustrate, let's make an analogy. You can liken your body in many ways to a car. When a hinge on a car door rusts it oxidizes. The logical solution would be to put oil on it. All oils have anti-oxidant properties. Many anti-oxidants (Like vitamins A or E) are oily and (in effect) do the same thing for your muscles that WD 40 does for the door hinge. It lubricates them, makes them more flexible, and allows them to retain oxygen for longer periods of time. Oxygen is a vital part of all body processes and especially tissue repair. As you grow older your body begins to lose the ability to retain oxygen in its tissues. Anti-oxidants help hold oxygen in your body's tissues at the cellular level, thereby slowing the aging process. This is why it's not unusual to find anti-oxidants listed as ingredients in skin and hair care products. Studies have also shown that supplementation with anti-oxidants can decrease the probability of cancer and increase lifespan.

It should be mentioned that oxygen can be damaging when present in an unstable form. Free radicals are actually toxic molecules of oxygen that adhere to and kill cellular compounds. Anti-oxidant supplements prevent free radical damage in your body that come from things like fatty fried foods, coffee, pesticides, sunlight, radiation, chemicals, pollution, cigarettes, alcohol, and petroleum-based products. In fact, the majority (close to 99%) of problems of the human body can be traced to a lack of stable oxygen in the tissues. These problems can be combated with common anti-oxidants such as vitamins A, C, D, and E, beta-carotene, flavinoids, pycnogenal, selenium, sulfur-containing amino acids, wheat germ oil, zinc, and herbs such as chamomile, echinacea, germanium, gingko, golden seal, milk thistle, and rosemary. These same anti-oxidants should be taken even after you are healed. Let's begin our supplements discussion by separating them into three groups: **vitamins**, **minerals**, and **other supplements**.

<u>Vitamins</u> facilitate tissue building/repair and are involved in the process of releasing energy (although they don't supply energy). Keep vitamins in a dark, cool (not cold) place as they are sensitive to air, heat, humidity and light. A shelf in a cupboard works fine. Additionally, certain vitamins (like A and D) will accumulate in your body and shouldn't be taken in excess. Other vitamins (like B and C) aren't stored in your body tissues (they're water soluble) and should be added to your diet. Whole grains and vegetables are generally a great source of vitamins and the skin of some vegetables (like potatoes) contains a lot of vitamins.

Vitamin A/Beta-carotene: The best kind of vitamin A is in liquid form (very oily). I prefer the gel capsules. Vitamin A is the "thinnest" oil. This could be compared to the viscosity ratings on engine oil. A is actually a thinner "viscosity" than vitamin E and therefore enters your system easier and faster. Deep yellow vegetables usually contain vitamin A in large amounts. Vitamin A also helps fight colds and flus (especially when zinc is taken as well). Beta-carotene is usually found in green leafy vegetables. Carotenes have been connected to life expectancy.

It should be mentioned that beta-carotene is not synonymous with vitamin A; beta-carotene is only one type of carotene. Vitamin A only contains certain types of carotenoids (like beta-carotene). Some carotenes not found in vitamin A have more anti-oxidant qualities and are deposited in the tissues in higher quantities. This is why eating a broad range of foods with high carotenoid levels is recommended. These include foods like berries, carrots, green leafy vegetables, plums, red cabbage, spinach, sweet potatoes, tomatoes, and yams. I take about 25,000 IUs of vitamin A daily (made from fish liver). Never take more than 150,000 IUs of vitamin A as this has been shown to damage the body.

The Vitamin B Complex: Take the B complex with meals. B12 is a great stress reducer. B6 is recommended for carpal tunnel syndrome (a minimum of 100 mgs. daily of B6). You should especially take the B complex if you play in smoky nightclubs. Never take the B complex with vitamin C-they will negate each other since the B complex is an alkaline and vitamin C is an acid. Great natural sources of the B complex include bananas, bran, brewer's yeast, broccoli, green leafy vegetables, kale, parsley, peanuts, spinach, tomatoes, wheat germ, and whole grains. Include some of these in your meals every day. I take the 150 mg. complex daily.

Vitamin C: Vitamin C is an acid that prepares collagen necessary for tissue repair. It's an anti-oxidant that is extremely important in any healing process. Take vitamin C with bioflavonoids in it-at least 5000 mgs. a day for tissue repair, and preferably Ester-C since it's designed to be absorbed by your body without acidifying. Additionally, rosehips are great because they're not synthetic. I used to take 10,000 mgs. daily when I started (5000 in the morning, 5000 in the evening). It's best to take vitamin C when you first wake up in the morning or before you go to bed at night on an empty stomach since it could acidify if combined with other foods. Other benefits of an increased vitamin C intake include a reduced risk of cancer, an increased lifespan, a reduction of LDL's (the bad cholesterol) in your body with a corresponding rise in HDL's (good cholesterol), and a more efficient immune system (due to the fact that vitamin C-rich foods produce the interferon that aids your body's immune system). Natural vitamin C is much better than a synthetic vitamin C. One orange has been said to be the equivalent of 10 grams of a synthetic C. Be sure to eat the stringy parts of fruits and vegetables close to the rinds since they tend to have the highest amount of bioflavonoids.

Use a stainless steel knife when cutting vitamin C-rich fruits and vegetables as black iron negates the beneficial effects of vitamin C. Citrus fruits are typically the best for vitamin C and bioflavonoids but many vegetables contain high amounts of these as well. Some of the best foods for vitamin C and bioflavonoids include broccoli, brussels sprouts, cabbage, cantaloupes, cauliflower, grapefruits, green peppers, guavas, lemons, limes, mustard greens, oranges, papayas, parsley, persimmon, raw leafy greens, red chili peppers, spinach, strawberries, tangerines, tomatoes, watercress, and white and sweet potatoes.

Bioflavonoids: These are anti-oxidants that have anti-inflammatory properties, increase your elasticity, prevent bruising, reduce the sodium content in your body, destroy free radicals, and are anti-carcinogenic and anti-viral. They can usually be found in darker fruits. Great natural sources of bioflavonoids include apples, blueberries, broccoli, cherries, cranberries, Hawthorne berries, onions, peaches, plums, and raspberries. I supplement my diet each day with a 1000 mg. bioflavonoid complex.

Vitamin D: This vitamin strengthens your bones and allows your body to utilize calcium. It's especially important to take D if arthritis runs in your family but be careful not to take too much as excessive doses can cause calcium to build up in your body. Natural sources of vitamin D include fruits, milk, nuts, the sun (your body will manufacture D when exposed to the sun), and vegetables.

Vitamin E: This is one of the "oils" that your "engine" (your body) requires. Most oils (like peanut oil) contain some vitamin E. E is an anti-oxidant that has anti-inflammatory properties, destroys free radicals, reduces the risk of cancer and cardiovascular diseases, helps increase elasticity, may repair digestive problems, and softens wrinkles. You should take 400 IUs for every ten years of your life; i.e., if you are 30 years old you should be taking 1200 IUs. Only take the natural vitamin E labeled "d-alpha tocopherol acetate". Anything starting with "dl-alpha" is a synthetic. Take extra vitamin E if you eat junk foods and never take it with iron-one's an acid, the other's alkaline. Vitamin E also works best when taken with selenium (another anti-oxidant). Great natural sources of vitamin E include beets, carrots, celery, and whole grains.

Minerals turn carbohydrates and fats into usable energy, help synthesize muscle tissue, speed up metabolic processes, and monitor chemical reactions in the body. Some minerals help tight muscles relax and relieve pain. Minerals (and oils) are especially important when dealing with tendonitis problems. Excessive cracking and popping noises from joints usually means you need more minerals. You can lose a lot of minerals by immersing yourself in hot water for long periods of time (such as a Jacuzzi, hot shower, etc.). Saunas will also cause mineral loss. Good sources of minerals are fruits, legumes, green leafy vegetables, and whole grains. It's especially important to eat a lot of fruits and vegetables as the body most easily absorbs the minerals in these. As for supplements, the next most easily absorbed minerals are those that are colloidal minerals (in liquid form), closely followed by chelated minerals. The main minerals that positively affect overuse injuries are calcium, chromium, magnesium, potassium, and sodium.

Potassium: A high-potassium, low-sodium diet reduces the risk of cancer and cardiovascular diseases and may lower blood pressure as well as prevent certain forms of arthritis. A typical American consumes twice as much sodium as potassium. This can easily be remedied by eating lots of fruits and vegetables (many fruits and vegetables contain 50 times more potassium than sodium). Good natural sources of potassium include apples, apple cider vinegar, asparagus, avocados, bananas, figs, fish, green leafy vegetables, meats, oranges, potatoes (with skin), poultry, prunes, sun-dried apricots, and whole grains.

Sodium is commonly found in salt but other products, such as baking powder or baking soda, also contain high amounts of sodium. Salt causes you to "rust"-just like saltwater causes rust on a car maintained in a beach area, salt is very corrosive and speeds the aging of the body as well as thickens the blood. To prevent the "rusting", you must use "oil"-take more vitamin E so your muscles don't get stiff.

Calcium: Calcium prevents muscle cramping but should be taken with vitamin D so it doesn't free-flow in your bloodstream (vitamin D keeps the calcium in your bones). Magnesium and potassium should also be taken with calcium as it's necessary for the proper utilization of calcium. The most widely known sources of calcium are dairy products (cheese, milk, yogurt, etc.), but did you know that some vegetables (particularly the dark green leafy type) have extremely high calcium levels as well? Vegetables like turnip greens, spinach, parsley, carrots, and broccoli are excellent sources of calcium. Other good natural sources of calcium are brewer's yeast, sunflower seeds, Brazil nuts, and almonds. Many professionals in the medical community believe that an adequate calcium intake combined with exercise can prevent osteoporosis, bone spurs and arthritis as well as lower blood pressure. I take a calcium/magnesium supplement daily-1000 mgs. calcium carbonate with 500 mgs. magnesium. Be sure to take the metallic calcium type with boron for maximum benefits.

Magnesium: Magnesium helps oxygen, vitamins, minerals, and nutrients get into your cells, facilitates the removal of waste products from your cells, may lower blood pressure, and is good for ligaments and tendons as it makes them supple and gives them more elasticity. You might say that magnesium allows your cells to eat and excrete, open and close. In effect, your cells breathe with magnesium. You can compare it to an engine-cleaning or carburetor-cleaning formula for your car: it facilitates easier passage through the system. Magnesium is best synthesized when present in chlorophyll from plants (especially dark green leafy vegetables). Other good sources of magnesium include dried beans and peas, whole grains, seeds, and nuts. It should be mentioned that vitamin and mineral supplements won't help much if you don't take magnesium.

Chromium: Chromium deals with blood sugar levels in the body. It allows the body's muscles to utilize insulin for energy. Unburned sugars in your blood get converted into fat and lactic acid without chromium. The result is that your muscles become tired easier (increasing your chances of injury), you become fatter, and lactic acid accumulates around already damaged tissues, impeding repair. Exercise exacerbates the problem. A lack of chromium may also cause a low blood sugar condition known as "Pica", a state where an individual craves sugar constantly. Good chromium sources include brewer's yeast and meat.

Other supplements help overuse injuries as well. Things like barley grass, chlorophyll, Coenzyme Q10, gelatin, ginkgo biloba, lecithin, Saint John's wort and shark cartilage have beneficial properties that enable overuse injuries to heal faster. I suggest trying each of them separately for a while and see if they have any effect on you. If they seem to be beneficial, add them to your list of treatments.

Barley grass: Barley grass is a great source of nutrients helpful to overuse injuries. It contains high quantities of beta-carotene, much of the B complex, vitamin C, calcium, chlorophyll, iron, magnesium, manganese, potassium, and zinc. Try the powder also. You can mix it in juice if you like.

Chlorophyll: Chlorophyll is an amazing product. I have had personal experience with it and can honestly say it has worked wonders for me as well as many other people I know. Medical studies have shown that chlorophyll has beneficial effects on inflammatory problems, wounds, and helps prevent cancer. Chlorophyll exists in plants but is found in higher concentrations in wheat grass, barley grass, spirulina, chlorella, and alfalfa. Other natural sources include spinach, parsley, lettuce and kale.

You can also buy chlorophyll in concentrated extract form. It is important to buy the right brand as processing methods vary and will consequently affect the results it has on you. The brand I always recommend is "DeSouza's" chlorophyll. Buy the 1 pint bottle and drink a bottle a day for three days. The reason for three days is that it takes that long for the body to get used to changes on a perfect PH (and chlorophyll has a perfect PH). In three days it'll either work or it won't. It basically de-toxifies your system as no disease can continually survive in a perfect PH. Chlorophyll is <u>loaded</u> with magnesium. If you find that it helps after three days you can try reducing your intake to the recommendation on the bottle and add 3 or 4 chlorophyll-rich alfalfa tablets each day.

Coenzyme Q10: Coenzyme Q10 allows our body's cells to release their own energy through the digestion or burning of food. This is required for daily tasks as well as the assimilation of nutrients, excreting waste products, and cellular reproduction. ATP (adenosine triphosphate) is created from this food burning and is how your body gets its energy. ATP is required on a regular basis as your body doesn't store much of it at any given time and must constantly be replenished. Coenzyme Q10 assists in the manufacturing of ATP. It essentially helps create energy for your muscles, boosting overall energy levels necessary for performance. Other benefits include helping the immune system as well as having anti-oxidant and anti-aging properties. It exists naturally in meats (organ meats particularly) as well as in broccoli, sesame oil, soy products, spinach, and wheat germ. Coenzyme Q10 is easily destroyed by cooking so care should be taken not to cook vegetables containing it.

Gelatin: Gelatin is essential for overuse injuries and is manufactured from the tendons and ligaments of animals. The concept is to replace your damaged tissues with similar types of tissues. Animal tendons and ligaments are about as close to your own tendons and ligaments as you are going to get. There is a product on the market called "Ligaplex 2" which supplies many of the nutrients available in gelatin but the cost is substantially higher, so gelatin is probably the most cost-effective way to go. A similar product, "Knox NutraJoint", is a gelatin product that also contains vitamin C and calcium. It is also very expensive and I cannot attest to the benefits of it as I do not suffer from overuse pain anymore. I therefore still recommend "Knox Unflavored Gelatin". You can purchase "Knox Unflavored Gelatin" in virtually any supermarket. Take a half package of the gelatin when you wake up and another half package before you go to sleep. I usually take it alone (it makes your mouth gummy), but if you don't like this method you can always mix it in a fruit juice drink.

Ginkgo-biloba: Ginkgo-biloba is known for its role in improving circulation and oxygenation of the tissues as well as building a strong cardiovascular and immune system. Oxygenation of the tissues provides greater elasticity for the muscles and retards aging-it helps prevent your body from "rusting".

Lecithin: Lecithin cleans up wastes in your system (including lactic acid) by breaking wastes products up into smaller pieces for easier removal. This may be accomplished through the use of certain phosphatides contained in lecithin. It is basically a bloodstream/blood vessel cleanser. Other purported benefits include lessening the chances of atherosclerosis, memory improvement, and the removal of stones in the gall bladder. Lecithin can be purchased at any health food store and also exists naturally in egg whites. I add lecithin granules to my cereal but have found the taste so unnoticeable that I can add it to a variety of things.

Saint John's Wort: Saint John's Wort has anti-bacterial properties that help reduce inflammation in damaged areas. It also contains hypericin, which is a sedative that works on the nervous system to relieve anxiety, depression, hypertension, and stress. Other purported benefits include helping exterior wounds heal faster, alleviating respiratory disorders, and cleaning the kidneys.

Shark cartilage: Shark cartilage assists in rebuilding and repairing cartilage in damaged areas of the body. It does this by providing cartilage as building material. It also contains certain amino acids and complex carbohydrates that discourage new blood vessel formation in the body, thereby limiting inflammation and swelling in the damaged area. Other nutrients like chondroitin sulfate and mucopolysaccharides, besides being beneficial for joints and cartilage, also assist in keeping inflammation at bay. This in turn helps alleviate aches, pains, and stiffness and increases flexibility. It is highly touted as a treatment for arthritis and other degenerative bone and joint ailments. It should be taken for at least one month as the body needs this much time to become acclimated to it.

Other Notes: You may want to experiment with the times of day you take your supplements, keeping a log of how you feel so you can recognize a cause-and-effect relationship. As an example, I tried taking vitamins A and C with bioflavonoids just before sleeping and found I would wake up in the morning with slight muscular aggravation. I attributed this to the highly acidic nature of vitamin C and therefore changed my schedule so that I would take these vitamins in the morning and afternoon (which eliminated the problem).

DIET

The adage "you are what you eat" is especially true today. It's no wonder there's such a high incidence of heart disease, cancer, arthritis, overuse injuries, depression and fatigue when you consider the average American diet: artificial ingredients, fatty fried foods, meats filled with nitrates, preservatives, processed foods, refined sugar in just about everything (including toothpaste), and so on. A typical American diet is also lacking in many nutrients. Chromium, for example, is almost non-existent. Other nutrients not sufficiently provided for in the American diet include the B complex (especially vitamin B6), calcium, iron, magnesium, and zinc. This does more damage to your body than one would realize and has everything to do with overuse injuries. You may wonder how your diet could have an effect on overuse injuries. Let's discuss this in detail below.

You must provide your body with the correct tools it needs to be able to fix itself, those tools being enzymes, fiber, hormones, minerals, and vitamins. So where do these "tools" come from? Your diet. What should a nutrient-rich diet consist of? A good diet should be high in complex carbohydrates. At least 50 to 75% of your diet should be in the form of complex carbohydrates, available in raw foods like fruits, nuts, seeds, vegetables, and whole grains. Another 10 to 15% should come from protein sources, including red meat, chicken, fish, beans, nuts, and seeds. The remaining percentage can be in the form of refined carbohydrates and polyunsaturated fats. I try to avoid refined foods altogether. This is because refined foods (white flour, white sugar, alcohol, and dairy products) cause a multitude of problems that we'll discuss later.

In this section I will explain the effects different types of foods have on your body. Perhaps the best way to begin is to start with the four basic food groups: **meats, dairy products, vegetables/fruits, and breads/cereals**. It should be mentioned that foods from any of these groups are good for you when they are in their natural, unrefined/unprocessed state. The main point is that the food you eat should be *as close to the way it actually exists in nature as possible-*

unprocessed, unrefined, fresh, organic, whole. Remember that these are the "tools" your body needs for repair. Give it the good stuff. And try to be disciplined. Eating garbage foods may cause a recurrence of problems.

Meat: There is much in the news about the bad effects meat has on the body. Actually, what they say about meat is true-but only when you consume it in extraordinary amounts. Your body only requires about two 4½-ounce servings of meat a week. This is just a little bigger than a deck of cards. This must be lean red meat, however, as red meat is the closest to our own tissues and is the only meat that contains the proper amounts of necessary amino acids (with the correct RNA), including certain trace amino acids that are only found in meats. You want to replace your own damaged muscle tissues with muscle tissues that are as close to your own as possible.

It's good to realize there is a protein coating around every cell in your body and meat supplies that protein. Without meat in your diet a particular syndrome-"Dupuytren's disease"-occurs in some people; tendons and ligaments shorten since protein isn't available to repair them and pain is caused from the resulting pressure exacted on the nerve endings. Meats are also a great source of iron, chromium, and zinc. Avoid luncheon meats as they are often loaded with nitrates and preservatives. Fish is also good for you as it often contains many fatty acids beneficial to the body. Avoid too much shellfish, however, as they are bio-accumulators. Meats should be thought of in the same way as condiments-something to add to your food rather than the meal itself. Incidentally, don't overuse amino acid supplements as they put unnecessary strain on your liver.

Dairy products: Dairy products should be avoided. Milk and cream not only dilute stomach enzymes but coat the stomach as well, making it difficult to properly digest foods you eat. They are also difficult to digest themselves. Remember, a calf uses three stomachs to digest milk. Perhaps the best reason to cut out dairy products is that they impede the oxygenation of muscle tissues and other body processes due to their mucous-like consistency. They clog up your system and cause congestion. This is why doctors will often recommend refraining from dairy products when suffering from cardiovascular illnesses such as bronchitis and pneumonia.

Cheese retards the oxygenation of your body for the same reason. Its sticky, mucous-like qualities make it adhere to a dish-and this is what it does inside your body. Cheese also contains large amounts of salt, causing your blood to thicken. Because of this slowing of the oxygenation process it is recommended that injured people avoid dairy altogether. The exception is eggs (although four egg yolks or more in a week is not a good idea for cholesterol reasons).

Fresh fruits and vegetables: Fresh fruits and vegetables are probably the most beneficial of the four food groups. They contain high levels of vitamins, minerals, enzymes and other nutrients necessary to repair damaged tissues, are low in calories, high in fiber (so that you feel full, lose weight and clean the digestive tract), and contain no cholesterol. Many of the vegetables from the cabbage family (broccoli, Brussels sprouts, cabbage, cauliflower, and turnips) also have properties that lower the incidence of cancer. Green leafy vegetables (lettuce, spinach) are good for the lungs and may help prevent osteoporosis while dark green vegetables have high levels of vitamins A, B, and C and contain the minerals calcium, iron, and magnesium.

Remember to buy fresh vegetables. Canned or frozen vegetables offer little nutritional value and often have preservatives, butter or cream added. Fresh fruits are also recommended. Eat the pulp and skin when you can since they are usually a good source of vitamins. You might want to shop on the day your grocer receives his produce so you'll know it's fresh. While both fruits and vegetables are good for you, try to lean more towards vegetables than fruits. An average American diet has a high acid content. Since fruits are generally more acidic while vegetables are typically alkaline, eating more vegetables helps to level out the acid/alkaline balance in your system. It should be mentioned that some people have allergies to "nightshade" vegetables (bell peppers, eggplant, potatoes, and tomatoes), which reportedly may increase inflammation. It's a good idea to avoid them if you notice your muscles aching more when you consume them.

Unrefined breads and cereals: Unrefined breads and cereals provide a variety of benefits-energy provided by complex carbohydrates, living enzymes and hormones, minerals and vitamins. Weight loss is another benefit as these foods have plenty of fiber that makes you feel full without putting on calories.

It is important to eat underlined breads and cereals as almost all of the aforementioned items-enzymes, fiber, hormones, minerals, and vitamins-are either removed or destroyed completely in the refining process. For example, almost 100% of the B6 vitamin (known to help carpal tunnel syndrome) is destroyed when breads and cereals are refined. They are refined for shelf life purposes but are essentially dead foods as the life has been destroyed or removed from them. This is why they last so long without going stale or molding. White flour products are also hard on your liver and gall bladder. Avoid them. I prefer the taste of whole grains; hopefully you will too.

It should be mentioned that the body cannot exist without six essential nutrients. We will discuss each of these nutrients in turn as they pertain to overuse injuries and mention some other things that should be a part of your diet as well as a rehabilitative program. The six nutrients are:

1) **Carbohydrates**: Complex carbohydrates are necessary for energy and stamina. It's a good idea to load up on complex carbohydrates when you are physically active or perform for long periods of time. Why must they be *complex* carbohydrates? The answer is in the structure of a complex carbohydrate. It's constructed from longer strings of simple sugars and carbohydrates. Since the body has to break these strings down into smaller carbohydrates and sugars (through digestion) before they can be utilized, complex carbohydrates provide a steady, time-released energy source. Complex carbohydrates are found in vegetables and whole grains.

Be aware that problems can also be caused by over-ingestion of complex carbohydrates. They can retard the oxygenation of your tissues due to the amount of unused energy that remains in your system. I find myself looser and pain-free when I stop eating after 6:00 P.M. since my body has used up most of the energy provided by complex carbohydrates ingested earlier. Find a happy medium.

2) **Fats**: Although a reviled topic in our culture, fats are absolutely necessary (hence the term "essential fatty acids"). It's saturated fat and cholesterol you want to avoid (due to problems with absorption by the body). Polyunsaturated fats and oils, on the other hand, provide a myriad of benefits. They carry a variety of beneficial nutrients to the cells in your body such as vitamins A, D, E, and K as well as gamma-linoleic acid (an essential fatty acid), used by your system for cellular repair; they improve flexibility; they coat the joints in your system, making it more difficult for acids to aggravate them (acids like vitamin C); and most importantly, they retard the oxidizing of the tissues. Other benefits include relief from dry skin, constipation, and younger-looking skin.

Beneficial sources of fats include borage, canola, evening primrose, flaxseed, olive (extra virgin), peanut, rosehip, safflower, sesame seed, and wheat germ oils. You may have noticed many of these oils are used in anti-aging and skin care products to reduce the signs of aging. The anti-oxidant properties that reduce signs of aging ("rusting") also lubricate and oxygenate damaged tissues. A muscle resists healing when it's dry and therefore needs to be oiled. You should also switch oils frequently to insure you are getting a variety of benefits. I take a variety of oils and put them in a row (from closest to furthest) in the cupboard, moving the closest one to the furthest position from me after use.

3) **Minerals**: Minerals are essential as previously mentioned in the "Supplements" section.

4) **Proteins**: Proteins are necessary for the building of body tissues. Although many foods supply protein, only red meat (from cows/buffalo/venison) provides all the amino acids in the proper amounts with the correct RNA. Eggs, fish, fruits and vegetables, grains, and poultry are good protein sources but are *incomplete* proteins since they don't supply all the amino acids in the required amounts. *Any serious treatment program for overuse injuries must involve the consumption of red meat!* Vitamin B6 is also necessary to properly utilize proteins. Avoid combining proteins with refined carbohydrates as it's hard on your system. Finally, don't eat excessive amounts of protein as it's hard to digest. The average person needs only two 4½-ounce servings of meat a week. Take a little more if you exercise.

5) **Vitamins**: Vitamins were discussed previously in the "Supplements" section.

6) **Water**: Water is necessary to our basic survival and assists in transporting nutrients in and waste products out of all cells in the body. Drink a certain amount of water each day without it being a part of something else. Your body considers fruit juice to be a food, for example, so it basically digests it as a food, not as water (even though it contains water). How much do you need? You probably shouldn't drink more than 8 glasses a day. More than this on a consistent basis might cause light-headedness due to the lowering of blood sugar levels.

Special consideration should be given here pertaining to certain foods, dietary additives, and nutrients when discussing any recuperative dietary program:

Alcohol is a refined food and as such should not be consumed. The detrimental effects of alcohol are well documented and certain characteristics of it affect overuse injury recovery time. Alcohol is devoid of most nutrients (enzymes, fiber, hormones, minerals, and vitamins) and most alcoholic drinks contain large amounts of sugars. It's best to completely remove alcohol from your diet.

Apples contain pectin (see below), ellagic acid and glutathione. Ellagic acid is an antioxidant that may also help to prevent cancer. Another antioxidant/body detoxifier and cancer-fighting substance is glutathione. All of these substances are found in fresh apples and apple juice (avoid processed apple juice). As is the case with all antioxidants, these substances speed the tissue repair and rebuilding process.

Caffeine should be avoided as it causes your blood vessels to constrict, thereby limiting blood flow to all areas of the body. Your blood carries oxygen to damaged tissues, which aids in the repair process. Other effects of caffeine include feeling worn down when you "crash" and disturbing sleep patterns when consumed late at night.

Enzymes are catalysts. When consumed with vitamins they cause the quickening or retarding of all sorts of important chemical reactions within the body, including reparative work and cellular construction. If enzymes are contained in the foods we eat, less of the body's own enzymes will be used to digest them, allowing the extra energy saved from digestion to be diverted elsewhere (like reparative work). Live enzymes are the key and can only be found in living foods. **Nothing bottled or canned has enzymes.** The enzymes in canned or bottled foods are destroyed in the canning or bottling process so they can have a long shelf life. Fruits and vegetables are a great source of enzymes. Some of the most beneficial enzyme sources are asparagus, broccoli, cabbage, carrots, parsley, papaya, squash, Swiss chard, and watercress.

Fiber keeps you regular, lowers the incidence of cancer by keeping foods from lingering in the intestinal tract, and helps you lose weight by making you feel full sooner. Fiber is great for mineral absorption and some types of fiber (known as lignans) have antioxidant properties. Unprocessed and unrefined fruits, grains, and vegetables are the best sources of fiber. Vegetables with the highest fiber content are the crunchy ones (carrots, potatoes, and so on). Eat the skin also as it contains a lot of fiber (fruits too). Don't overlook beans and peas as many are excellent sources of fiber. Good choices include black, garbanzo, lima, kidney, and green beans as well as black-eyed, green, and split peas.

Garlic aids the system with the removal of waste products and cleans blockages from the bloodstream by dilating blood vessels. It also helps lower blood pressure levels. Raw garlic is recommended which can be added to a homemade salad dressing.

Pectin assists in building cartilage as well as neutralizing wastes in the body. It also lowers cholesterol and builds strong fingernails. The best source of pectin is in apples where it is concentrated in the skin. Other sources include avocados, bananas, cherries, grapes, peaches, pineapples, raisins, raspberries, and tomatoes.

Prostaglandins are hormones made by the body's cells. These hormones govern many body processes including anti-inflammatory responses. Foods like canola oil, cod liver oil, flaxseed oil and onions are utilized by the cells in the production of prostaglandin, which helps keep inflammation at bay.

Salt speeds the "rusting" process of your body. One could make an analogy between a car stored near a salt-water environment and our own bodies. The result is the same. Rust is oxidation (not to be confused with oxygenation); metal oxidizes or loses the ability to retain oxygen. In a similar way, this is what happens to the body when excessive salt is ingested (easy to do on the typical American diet). Salt is also hard on your gall bladder. Salt is necessary but may be obtained in sufficient amounts from whole, unrefined foods. I don't keep salt in my home and prefer seasoning my food with garlic, garlic powder, lemon juice, "Mrs. Dash" (a salt-free seasoning), onion powder, olive oil and apple cider vinegar along with herbs and spices.

Sugar is extremely detrimental to the overuse injury recovery process. Like white flour, white sugar is refined for shelf life purposes; sugar cane or sugar beet juice would go bad quickly otherwise. The enzymes, fiber, hormones, minerals, and vitamins are removed in the refining process while energy is extraordinarily concentrated, resulting in a concoction that is too strong for the body to cope with adequately. This is like using nitro-methane in a factory built car. White sugar shuts down the natural cortisone in your body responsible for reparative work. In addition, tendons or ligaments may become tight and inelastic due to the absence of necessary oils in the system. This absence is brought about by pancreatitis-a common problem with people who consume high amounts of sugars. Enzymes from your pancreas produce specific types of alcohols that break down the body's oils. Chocolate is the worst. When chocolate is consumed the body loses large amounts of important minerals and cannot assimilate calcium for a day or more. It might be said that chocolate is a "de-mineralizer". Brown sugar is easier on the system than white sugar and honey is better than brown sugar; however, it is recommended that sugar is avoided as much as possible if not altogether. Typical products to avoid include cakes, candy, cereals with sugar added, chocolate, cookies, donuts, ice cream, jams and jellies, pies, and soft drinks. Many other products such as alcohol, bacon, cigarettes, fruit drinks, potato chips, salt, and toothpaste also often contain sugar.

How can one be sure that they're not getting added sugar? Read the labels. Avoid products containing obvious sugars stated in the ingredients as well as ingredients ending with the letters "ose": dextrose, fructose, glucose, lactose, and sucrose are common examples. Other products containing large amounts of sugars are fruit juice concentrates (concentrated apple juice) and syrups (like corn syrup). Avoid synthetic sugars like sucralose, aspartame, Splenda and Nutrasweet. Also remember that excessive sugar intake from any source-even natural fruits and fruit juices-can be detrimental, so use these moderately. If you do eat high sugar foods, your body will assimilate them better if they are consumed on an empty stomach. It has been purported that combining higher sugar foods with higher protein foods (like a steak with wine or grape juice) is not a good idea. I personally haven't noticed any bad effects when combining unrefined sugars and proteins in non-excessive amounts but your experience may be different than mine. Incidentally, an excessive desire for sweets is typically caused by a lack of complex carbohydrates, a lack of adequate protein, or insufficient chromium intake.

Wheat germ speeds waste elimination and body repair times, provides fiber, and has antioxidant properties (through the component known as octacosanol). The fiber in wheat germ is of the lignan variety. Wheat germ contains high amounts of vitamin B6 and beneficial fatty acids.

To sum up: unrefined foods should constitute the overwhelming majority of your diet. Refined foods (alcohol, dairy products, white flour and white sugar) should be a very small part of your diet (if not avoided altogether). In the case of alcohol, white flour, and white sugar, these foods should be avoided as they are lacking in essential enzymes, fiber, hormones, minerals, and vitamins that are required for tissue repair. In addition, what's left behind is a very rich, concentrated concoction of pure energy that your body ultimately can't handle. This energy is ultimately converted into fat or lactic acid if not burned off through heavy exercise immediately afterwards. Lactic acid not only irritates inflamed or damaged areas but can also accumulate in these areas, impeding blood flow and oxygenation. Dairy products impede the oxygenation of muscle tissues and other body processes due to their mucous nature. Some of these foods may cause blockages in the intestines, producing other problems. Dietary discipline is an obvious requirement when trying to recover from or prevent overuse injuries. Your diet has everything to do with the way you feel. Increased energy will result from a diet following these guidelines.

Many health food markets carry products that are healthy alternatives. All natural, unrefined foods choices such as vegetarian chorizo (without nitrates) and mayonnaise (without dairy or sugar) are available. A creative person can use these products to come up with many delicious meal ideas-an example might be to mix mustard with spices into some all-natural mayonnaise to make a dip for vegetables such as bell peppers, carrots, green beans, radishes and raw squash.

Another example might be chorizo sandwiches with all-natural mayonnaise, mustard, romaine lettuce, and whole grain bread. Being creative with healthy foods will make an easier transition to a good diet so you don't feel like you're missing out.

COOKING

Care should be taken when cooking to receive the maximum benefits that foods have to offer. Many vitamins are sensitive to cooking methods. Fried vegetables lose approximately 70% of the B6 vitamin while boiling inactivates 50% of the vitamin C content and steaming inactivates 30% of the vitamin C content. Vegetables should not be cooked longer than necessary. The shorter the cooking time the better. The best choice is not to cook them at all but many people find this to be an unpleasant alternative. These people may find that unsavory raw vegetables are more easily swallowed as a juice (see below).

Since cooking seems to be a necessity for many, keep these points in mind:

(1) Wash your vegetables quickly as many vitamins are destroyed by water (especially vitamin C). Soaking is not recommended. Direct light, heat, drying, and aging can also destroy vitamins. Get <u>fresh</u> foods and store them in airtight containers in a dark drawer in the refrigerator. Avoid cutting them until you are ready to eat them.

(2) The least damaging cooking methods are steaming, simmering, poaching, cooking in it's own broth/juice or stewing, roasting, baking, stir-frying, and boiling. These cooking methods should be remembered not only at home but when dining at a restaurant as well. Of course, "garden fresh" is the best description your food should have. Always try to consume live foods-by "live" I mean that the food becomes old or moldy very quickly and usually must be kept in the refrigerator to prolong its life. Live foods are always the best choice-refined or processed foods are basically dead (which is why they have a long shelf life). You want to replace damaged muscle tissues with healthy living tissues, so try not to cook your food too much (if at all).

JUICING

Humans initially started out as hunter/gatherers and ate enormous amounts of raw foods. Evolutionarily speaking, our bodies have adapted to a primarily raw food diet. In today's world most us don't eat the same amount of raw food as our ancestors. Juicing makes it possible for us to get the benefits of eating large amounts of raw food every day without the bulk. This is especially important if you don't really care for the taste of raw foods like broccoli-you can cover up the taste of broccoli by adding carrots or apples. You get all the benefits of the vegetables (except for fiber) from the juice. Juicing is also easier on your digestive system and is absorbed quicker since the body doesn't require much digestive effort. In fact, juicing might even be better than eating raw fruits and vegetables as it practically guarantees nutrient absorption since they're broken down into an easily digested liquid. All beneficial nutrients are in a concentrated but balanced form that oxygenates the body and speeds reparative and cleansing processes. Furthermore, when you juice at home you know what you're getting - most commercial fruit and/or vegetable drinks have added sugar or salt.

In this section we will discuss juicing and juice combinations that help overuse injuries as well as specific benefits certain juices give you. Here are some things to consider before we begin. Keep all fruits and vegetables in your refrigerator until you're ready to juice them. Cut them only when you're ready to begin juicing and avoid using an iron knife as it could destroy the vitamin C in foods (I use a stainless steel knife).

Try to drink the juice within a minute of juicing the fruits/vegetables. Have you ever seen the inside of an apple turn brown after you cut it open? The enzymes begin to die and this is what happens when you juice fruits and vegetables. It's important to get those live enzymes inside you quickly while they are still active.

Try to drink your juice before meals. Lean towards vegetable juices more than fruit juices. While fruit juices are more palatable and do contain many good nutrients, they almost always contain high amounts of sugars and as such should not be over ingested. They are also usually more acidic than alkaline, and since the typical American diet is highly acidic it's a good idea to lean more towards vegetables. In fact, a good rule of thumb is that vegetables are usually alkaline while fruits are usually acidic. Finally, try to avoid mixing fruits with vegetables when juicing. Now let's talk a little about various juices and combinations and how they may be beneficial to you:

Apple juice contains high levels of pectin, ellagic acid and glutathione. These substances help speed tissue repair and rebuilding. Other benefits include better elimination and possibly helping eradicate viruses from your system. A beneficial drink for overuse injuries is fresh apple juice with a half package of gelatin mixed in.

Apricot juice contains enzymes, hormones, minerals, and vitamins necessary for tissue repair and keeps the bloodstream clean.

Beet juice cleans many of the filtering organs in your body such as the kidneys. It also contains high amounts of the A and C vitamins and cleans your bloodstream and nervous system. This cleansing of the filtering organs provides for better waste disposal.

Blueberry juice contains high amounts of bioflavonoids necessary to properly utilize vitamin C.

Cabbage juice contains high amounts of beneficial enzymes, hormones, minerals, and vitamins. Other benefits include intestinal cleansing and possibly healing ulcers. Cabbage is part of the cruciferous vegetable group-a group of vegetables that is very high in nutrients. Other members of this group are asparagus, broccoli, Brussels sprouts, and cauliflower; all of these should be considered staples in any juicing program.

Carrot juice contains high amounts of vitamin A, an antioxidant. Other benefits include the cleansing of skin blemishes, the digestive system, and the ability to stay in the sun for longer periods of time without getting sunburned (due to vitamin A).

Celery juice is a blood purifier and also cleans up your kidneys and liver.

Cherry juice contains high levels of bioflavonoids.

Cranberry juice cleans impurities out of the blood and cleans the kidneys. Other benefits include preventing bladder and prostate gland problems and preventing flus.

Black or red currant juice contains many powerful organ-purifying properties. The nutrients in these juices clean up waste products that accumulate in the digestive organs. It should be a staple in your juicing program.

Pineapple juice contains high amounts of bromelain, a natural anti-inflammatory and pain reliever. Since the leaves contain the highest levels of bromelain, it is suggested that you juice them with the rest of the pineapple. In fact, juice the entire pineapple, skin and all. Pineapple is also high in beneficial nutrients and breaks down mucus in your system.

An **Apple-lemon-carrot juice mixture with gelatin** is a wonderful combination for overuse injuries. The apple provides pectin; the lemon provides bioflavonoids, detoxifies your system, and "recharges" your system since it is an anonic food (discussed later); carrot juice provides vitamin A; and gelatin is the raw material that your body uses to replace damaged tissues with.

Carrot-celery juice is good for keeping you from over-perspiring when you begin your exercise program. It also contains many beneficial nutrients.

One last juice that should be mentioned (although hardly ever juiced at home) is **aloe vera juice**. This juice can be picked up at any health food store and contains high amounts of vitamin C. It can be mixed in with fruit juice since its taste leaves something to be desired.

EATING HABITS

Besides dietary considerations, what about the process of eating itself? Are there proper eating "techniques" that ensure maximum assimilation of crucial nutrients necessary for tissue repair? How do you assure variety in your diet? When and how much should you eat? These and other related topics are discussed in this section, helping you make the transition from a poor diet to a good one easier. Remember your diet has everything to do with the way you feel, so your persistence will be rewarded. You are what you eat!

Let's begin with the actual **process of eating** itself. It's not a good idea to drink liquids with your meals. Liquids dilute the digestive enzymes in your stomach responsible for breaking down foods into readily assimilated nutrients. When these enzymes are diluted some of the food you eat goes to waste since many of the nutrients are lost to improper digestion. Instead of drinking with your meals, load up on liquids about 20-30 minutes <u>before</u> you eat. You can also wait until after you eat but be aware that it takes the body as much as two to three hours to properly digest some foods. It's better to drink before meals as liquids are assimilated quicker due to the minimal digestion necessary.

As far as solid foods, be sure to completely chew your food before swallowing. Remember that chewing is part of your body's digestive process; your saliva contains enzymes that help pre-digest food before it gets to your stomach. Europeans really have the right idea in this sense. Many countries in Europe treat dinner as a special social event that lasts for hours. Whereas Americans gulp down fast food in a matter of minutes, Europeans will sit down at a table for hours, relaxing and slowly savoring every bite while enjoying conversation with friends or family. This is the right idea. It's certainly a lot more enjoyable than popping a quick burger and fries in your mouth in front of the T.V. and your stomach will feel better afterwards. You may also find it enjoyable spending quality time with your spouse or children.

Regarding **variety**, it's obvious that eating one kind of vegetable exclusively will only expose you to the nutrients found in that vegetable. Eating a variety of foods assures maximum exposure to a wide range of nutrients. It also assures that nutrients not consumed on any given day will be consumed later in the week. It should be mentioned that certain foods-especially vegetables and other foods containing nutrients pertinent to overuse injuries-should make up the largest percentage of your diet. Keep the variety but lean heavily on these foods and food groups. In addition, ingesting nutrients from a variety of live foods is better than taking supplements as live foods contain living enzymes. It's recommended, however, that supplements be taken in addition to a good diet to assure you receive all necessary nutrients.

The easiest way to assure variety is to keep a journal. This may not sound appealing to those wishing to prevent overuse injuries. People currently suffering from chronic overuse problems, on the other hand, should seriously consider keeping a journal. In the journal, keep a record of what was eaten (to maintain variety in your diet); how you felt after you ate those foods (to see if there's a relationship with certain foods and how you feel); when you ate (to keep your system on a dietary schedule); what state of mind you were in when you slipped and went on a junk food binge (depressed?); and so on. The journal can also be used to record how you feel after trying various treatment methods or taking supplements; how much rest you are getting and whether you are on a consistent schedule; how you feel after exercising or stretching and your emotional states at the time; your overall attitude on any given day; and changes in playing or practicing techniques. By keeping a record you should see a correlation between changes you make in your lifestyle and how you feel. It will also show how poorly your body feels when you slip-up and go back to bad habits. This is powerfully reinforcing and will give you self-confidence and hope with the realization that you have the power to control how you feel.

You will slip-up occasionally. Everybody does, don't get depressed about it; rather, try to ascertain the reason you slipped. What was your emotional state? Did you miss a meal and felt justified to eat junk food since you hadn't eaten? Did you feel pressured into eating junk or refined foods since others around you were eating it? Where were you when you slipped?

Examine the surrounding circumstances when the slip-up occurred and make the required modifications so it doesn't happen again. Mistakes are an opportunity to learn.

As far as **when to eat**, do not eat any refined foods 4 to 6 hours before going to bed. Your body can't burn up the tremendous amount of refined energy before you retire so it gets converted into acids, glycogen, and fat. The acids formed go to damaged areas in the body and cause a variety of problems. Unless you're planning on jogging a couple of miles at midnight I would suggest following this rule. **This is one of the most important rules in this book.** Eating natural, organic foods as they are found in the wild like fruits, vegetables, and meats does not cause problems since the energy in them is not concentrated. I have found that having a big dinner made from natural foods usually sustains me for the rest of the evening. It also discourages weight gain.

This raises another question: **how much should you eat**? The amount will vary from person to person but the answer is the same-when you feel comfortably satisfied, that's when you should stop eating. It's estimated that it takes about 30 minutes to feel full after eating so eat until you're not hungry anymore, not until you feel full. Moderate food intake is the key. Insufficient food intake will deprive you of essential nutrients in sufficient quantities and cause a loss of muscle tissue and an inability to repair damaged tissues. Excessive food intake can cause acid, glycogen, fat, faster aging, and improper digestion of foods due to an inability of the stomach's enzymes to digest the large food quantities fast enough.

Since most people have problems with eating too much rather than too little, here are suggestions on how to deal with overeating. First, avoid eating between meals. Second, be sure you are actually hungry and don't just want to keep your mouth occupied or are eating to relieve stress. Third, adopt a meal schedule so your system becomes accustomed to eating at the same times each day. Fourth, save uneaten food for another meal if you're worried about it going to waste. Fifth, try exercising-exercise helps reduce hunger. Finally, stay busy. You won't be thinking about food if you're working hard. There have been days I've forgotten to eat because I was busy and realized I didn't eat at the day's end (not good). Incidentally, don't intentionally skip days for eating, but if you accidentally skip a day once in a while it is not so bad. It gives your stomach and your digestive system a rest and recuperative time.

One final thing you might want to try to make the transition from a bad diet to a good diet easier is to binge on junk food once a week as a reward for eating healthy the rest of the week. It's a good way to start your journey toward a better diet as it is positive reinforcement in two ways: 1) it rewards you for following your diet, and 2) it will show you a correlation between the food you eat and how it makes you feel. You may have more pain and muscular problems on binge days or the day after. You will also find that foods you used to enjoy will no longer be appealing to you the longer you remain on the diet. If you stop eating salt, chips will eventually taste too salty for you since your taste buds will have become more sensitive to flavors in foods. Your taste buds will become refined and you will not find it difficult to control your diet anymore.

CHAPTER 2:
MUSCLE CONDITIONING

Life has changed considerably since the 1900's. We use elevators instead of stairs, sit in front of computers, travel by car, buy pre-packaged foods at the supermarket, etc. There are benefits to our current comfort levels but it does have its price. The current sedentary lifestyle of most Americans creates many problems. These include overuse injuries. The key element in repairing damaged tissues-indeed, in repairing practically all of the body's problems-is oxygen. Oxygen not only prevents the "rusting" process, it is crucial for most chemical reactions in the body. These include reactions pertaining to brain functions, tissue repair and proper synthesis and use of foods. Aerobic exercise is the only type of exercise that delivers high amounts of oxygen to your bloodstream and is recommended over all other forms of exercise for overuse injuries. Aerobic exercise also causes your blood to circulate at a faster rate, speeding nutrients to damaged tissues while removing waste products quicker. Without aerobic exercise, the system begins to slow down; blood circulates slower, cells become starved for oxygen, chemical reactions occur less frequently, fewer nutrients are carried to damaged areas, and food not burned off through exercise gets converted to fat, glycogen, or acids.

Lactic acid in particular has a noticeable effect on overuse injuries. It's a by-product of excess glycogen. Glycogen causes lactic acid to crystallize in overused or injured areas. This is why you feel stiff or sore the day after a vigorous workout. When you sleep after exercise your circulation begins to slow down and lactic acid begins to settle in overworked areas. Lactic acid can become so concentrated in an area that it can drastically retard the healing process. Furthermore, the resultant aching from concentrated lactic acid can make you more prone to injury. This increase in stiffness and soreness is how your muscles tell you they are overworked and need more oxygen. Pain felt from overuse injuries is not actually from muscles themselves but from nerves in the damaged area. Lactic acid crystals are irritating and inflaming nerves, causing them to swell up and send pain messages to the brain. Lactic acid is often caused when muscles are worked hard but oxygen intake requirements are not met. What's needed is endurance, built by starting slow and gradually increasing the demands put on muscles through aerobic exercise. Lactic acid can be flushed from areas with massage, vibrating, stretching, and mild exercise. Let's begin our focus on muscle conditioning with a look at stretching.

STRETCHING

If you watch professional sports one thing becomes clearly evident: athletes stretch before playing. Athletes that don't begin their sport by stretching typically have short careers. As a musician I've learned to think of myself as an athlete. I never begin exercise, a long practice session, or a demanding job without stretching first. Returning to the car analogy, an engine lasts a lot longer if you let it warm up before you drive it. This can be said of our muscles. Muscles need to be warmed up before putting a load on them through stretching. It's also a good idea to warm down with stretching. Take a lesson from pro athletes and realize stretching should be a regular part of any lifestyle involving repetitive motion.

Stretching benefits muscles by:

• creating easier motions and greater agility from increased flexibility
• reducing the risk of muscular injuries (if done correctly)
• preparing your muscles for strenuous work
• helping you learn your body by making you more keenly aware of the muscles being stretched
• helping alleviate muscular (as well as psychological) tension
• oxygenating and nourishing muscles through increased blood flow/circulation to the stretched area

Incidentally, oxygen also makes your muscles more flexible. If you want proof, compare how flexible you are in the morning as opposed to the evening by stretching at both times. Notice your muscles are more flexible during evening stretches. This is because your body goes into a lower oxygen intake mode while sleeping. You are not as flexible in the morning after you wake because of this lowered intake. As the day goes on and you move and walk around your body requires more oxygen (explaining the increased flexibility in the evening).

We'll begin with the philosophies necessary to stretch correctly and how to find stretches that are helpful to you. The remainder of this section focuses on specific stretches helpful to overuse injuries.

Develop the proper attitudes toward stretching not only to gain the benefits but also to prevent further injury. Most people make the mistake of overstretching an injured area, compounding the injury. Cultivate the right attitude. You will become frustrated if you injure yourself by doing too much too soon, perhaps discouraging you to continue stretching. Don't worry if others are more flexible than you or you don't seem to be as flexible on a given day; people are genetically different and your body's flexibility will vary from day to day and times of day. Don't compete with others when stretching and be prepared for your body to be inconsistent. Some days will be tighter than others.

Stretching is a calm, tranquil thing, not forced. Be patient and relax. Don't have deadlines or make a contest out of it. Don't bounce. Be aware of how your body feels. Create a stretching schedule and be consistent with it, not just whenever you feel like it. Enjoy the stretch for its own sake, not worrying about being flexible. Flexibility will come at its own time. Don't try to force your muscles to do more than they should. Think of stretching as a non-event: you're intention is not to gain flexibility but to increase circulation and wake up your muscles. The real benefit will come from walking, swimming, or other exercises you do after stretching.

Enjoy the stretch for its own sake and always leave plenty of room to stretch more. You can make things worse if you don't as overstretching results in further damage to stretched areas. You will inevitably overstretch when you first begin stretching. When this happens take some time off, ingest more oils to lessen the damage, and learn from it by being more careful next time. With time you will gain flexibility if you stretch correctly on a daily basis.

Begin by slowly going into the stretch, find a comfortable (not strained) position where you feel a light pull, and hold it for half a minute. Notice your breathing. If your breathing is labored and quivering you are stretching too much. Ease up. You should be taking long, deep breaths to oxygenate the body while stretching. Take note of how the stretch feels to the muscles being stretched. While holding the stretch, learn to get in tune with your muscles and listen to them.

How do they feel? Is it a nice, relaxed stretch or a little too much? Find your thresholds and don't push too hard. Be aware of your body's limitations. Remember you are in control of how it feels. When doing a particular stretch, what other areas of your body seem to be affected? You will notice your muscles will begin to loosen up over the 30 seconds. Add another 15 seconds after this and stretch a little further, going for the feeling of a light pull once more. Your flexibility will vary at times so it is imperative to go slow and listen to your body. Slowly loosen up when releasing without any jerky fast motions. If you have pets, watch them. How do they stretch? A stretching pet's motions are non-competitive, slow, easy, relaxed motions that feel good. Got the picture?

Which stretches should you do? Since many muscle groups are interconnected, a tight, damaged muscle in one area may cause problems elsewhere by overextending a different muscle and putting excess pressure on it. This can lead to injury of that muscle as well. Hence, the optimum situation would be to do as many as you can fit in your schedule. Doing all stretches listed in this book may be unrealistic for some as busy schedules do not permit much free time. Therefore a good rule of thumb in choosing personal stretches is to find the ones that directly affect the injured area and its surrounding muscle groups. If your shoulder is giving you problems for example, find shoulder stretches that stretch out the specific injured muscles in your shoulder. Then do arm, elbow, and back stretches on that side of your body. It's also recommended to do the same stretches on the other side of your body to balance your muscles on both sides. Finally, if the stretches in this book don't seem to completely address your problem areas, experiment and try to find ones that do. Find stretches that directly affect the injured area and listen to your body. You should know your body better than anyone.

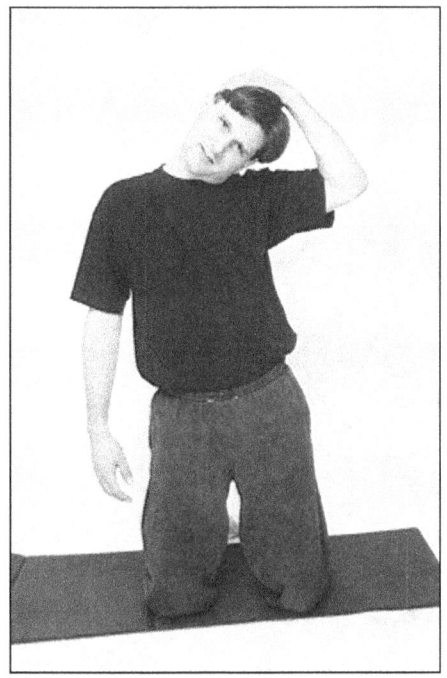

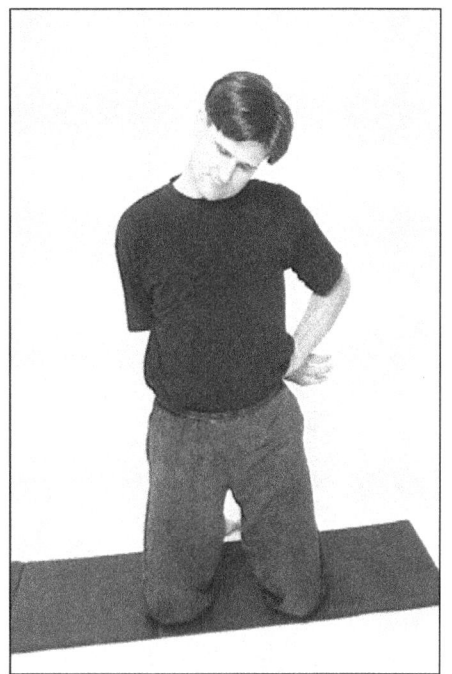

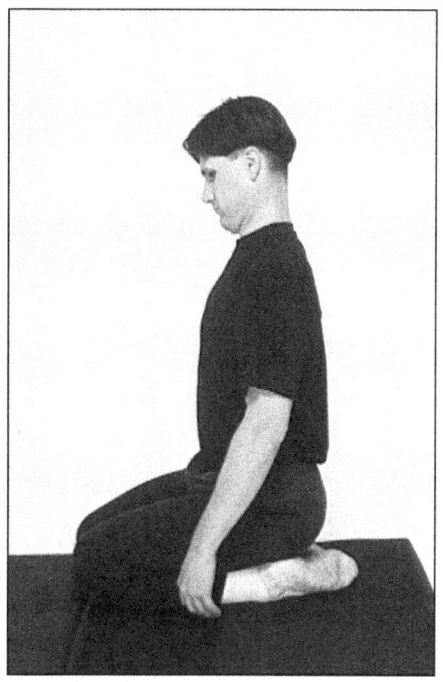

The following series of stretches are **neck stretches**. This particular stretch affects the side of the neck as well as the collarbone area. Be sure to stretch the other side too.

This stretch is similar to the previous one but affects the shoulder also. Pull your right hand toward your left side while leaning your head toward the left. Do both sides.

While keeping your shoulders to the back and down, try pointing the rear top area of your head to the ceiling. You should feel a pull in your collarbone area as well as the back of your neck.

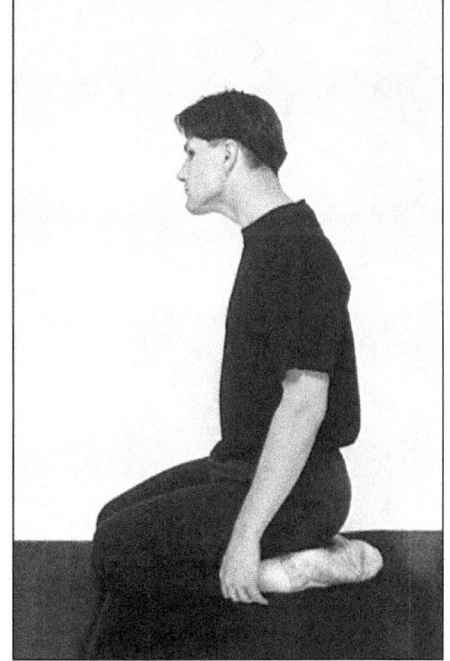

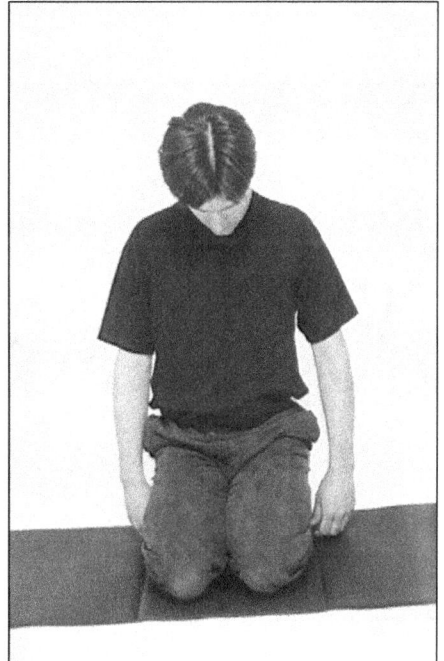

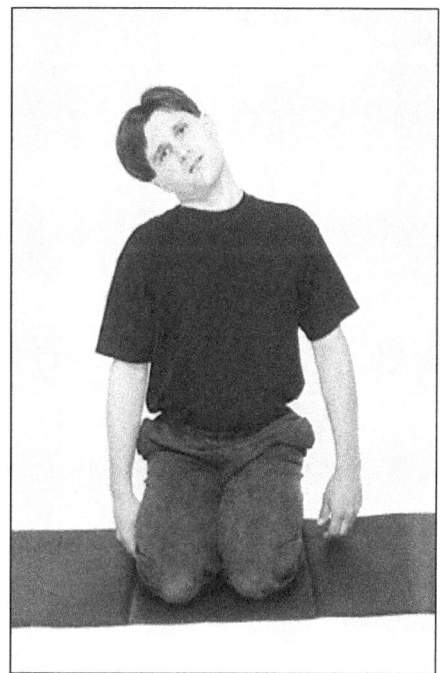

Push your chin out away from your body while keeping your shoulders to the back and down. You should feel a stretch in your collarbone, your back, and a little in the pecs.

This stretch rotates the head all the way around. Begin by letting your head hang down and slowly and gently push your head downward toward your groin as you loosen up.

After your neck loosens up, begin to rotate your head around by slowly rolling it to the right. Go as slow as you need to so all muscle groups are affected.

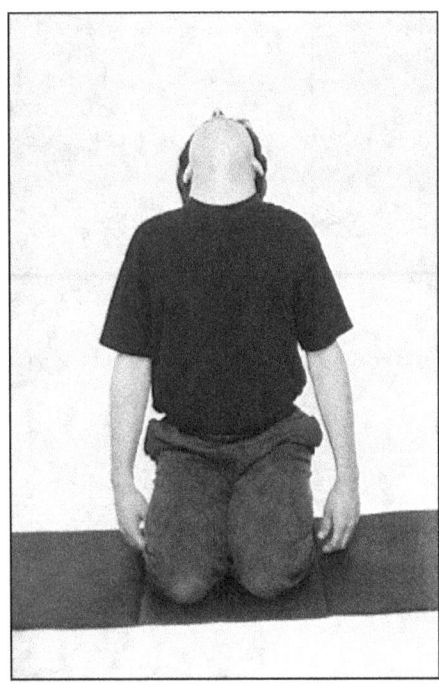

Continue with this stretch by slowly rotating your head towards your back. Again, go as slow as you need to and apply just enough pressure to get a nice, comfortable stretch.

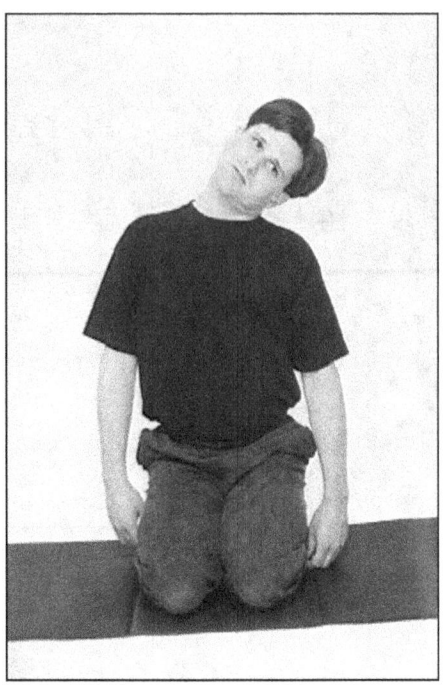

Slowly rotate your head to the left after completing the previous stretch. Be sure to go slow and stretch all muscle groups. Complete the circle by rotating your head to the front.

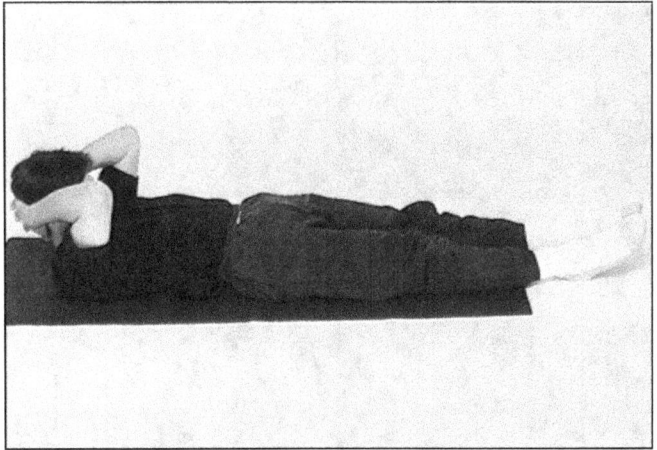

This particular stretch affects the back of the neck as well as the upper area of the back just below the neck. Apply even pressure with both hands and keep your head straight.

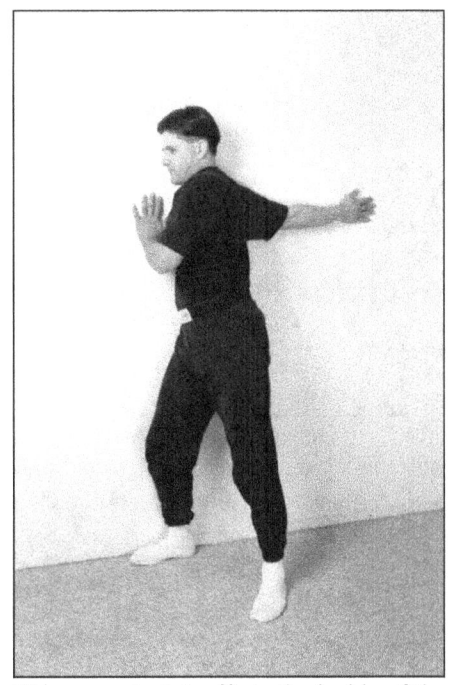

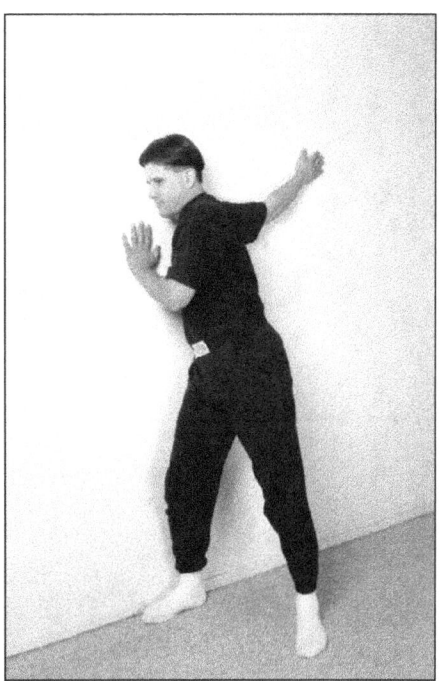

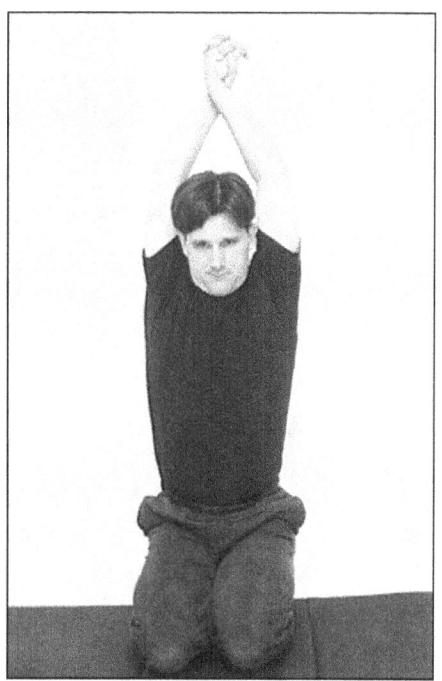

This **arm stretch** affects the inside of the arm all the way to the hand. Place the inside right shoulder to the wall and the right hand at a 90° angle to the body. Use your left hand to push away from the wall.

Continue the previous stretch by moving your arm up and down, thereby affecting the various muscles in your arm. Be sure to keep your shoulder to the wall. Continue by doing these first two arm stretches with the left arm.

On this stretch, clasp both of your hands together and push your hands upward towards the ceiling. This stretch affects the inside uppermost part of the arm as well as the outside of the armpit.

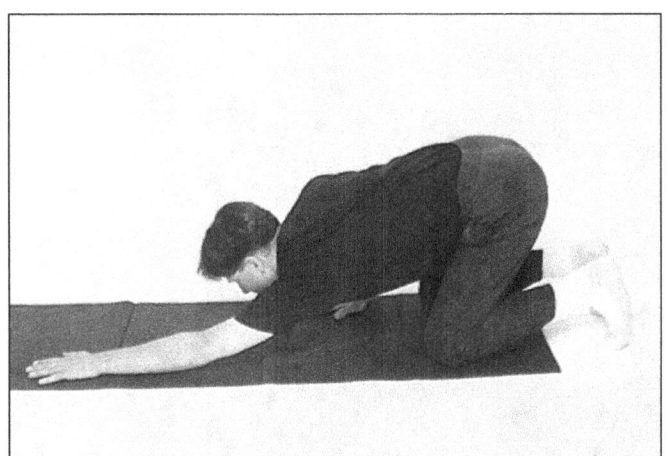

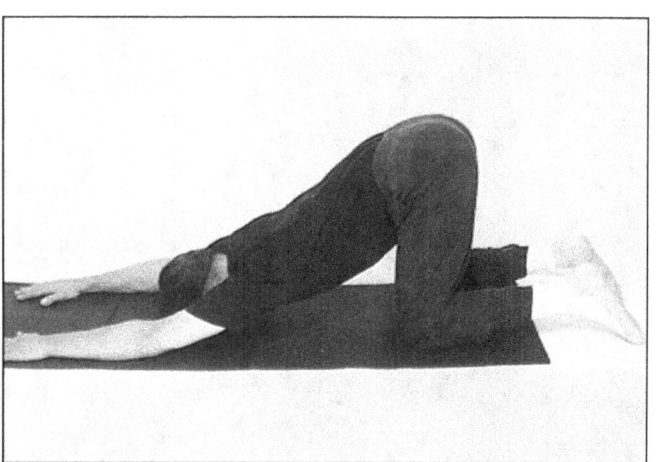

Stretch the underside of the arm, part of your shoulder, your lats, and upper back by firmly placing your hand on the floor and pulling back away from your hand. Be sure that your arm remains straight. Do the other arm as well.

Continue with the previous stretch by putting both hands on the floor at the same time, being sure to keep both arms straight. Affect different groups of muscles more or less by rocking from one side to the other.

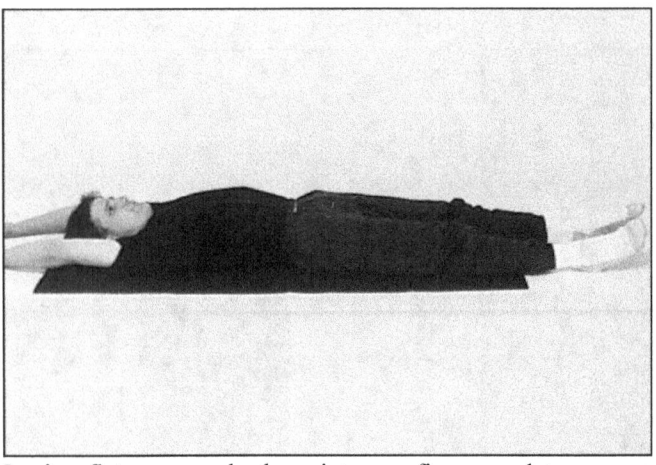

Laying flat on your back, point your fingers and toes away from your body, stretching not only your arms but also your sides and legs. Be sure to keep the arms and legs straight. Apply just enough pressure to achieve an easy, comfortable stretch.

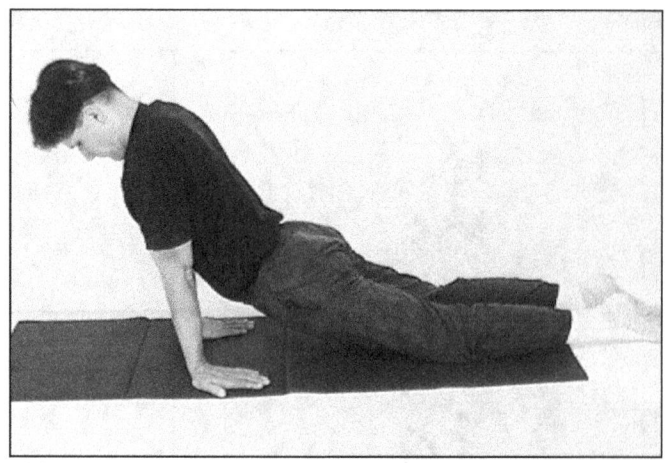

This series of **hand/wrist stretches** begins by placing your hands on the floor with your fingers toward your feet. While keeping the arms straight and your palms on the floor, slowly pull your shoulders back towards your feet.

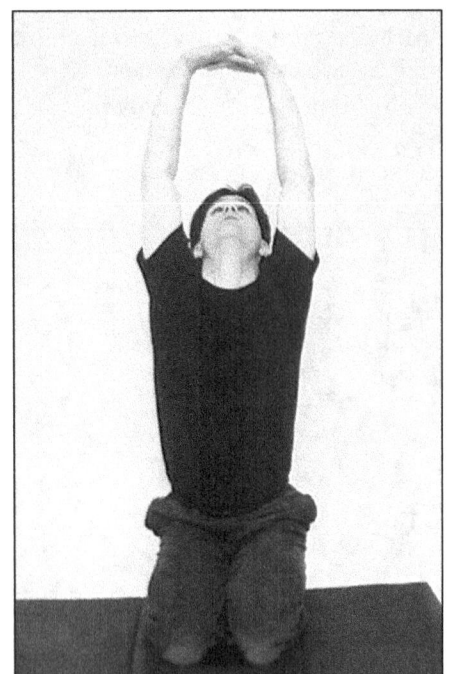

This stretch affects the inside of the wrist (including the carpal tunnel area), the lats, and the inside forearm. Clasp your hands together as shown and push the palms of your hands toward the ceiling.

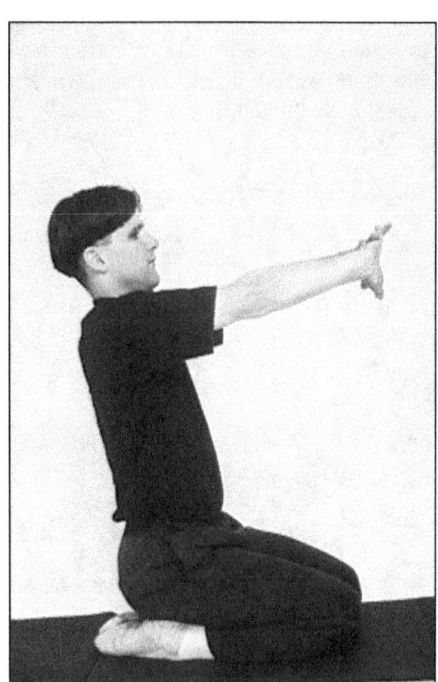

Continue the previous stretch by slowly moving your hands down in front of you, being sure to keep your palms directed outward and your arms straight. You can move your hands to the left or right to affect different areas more.

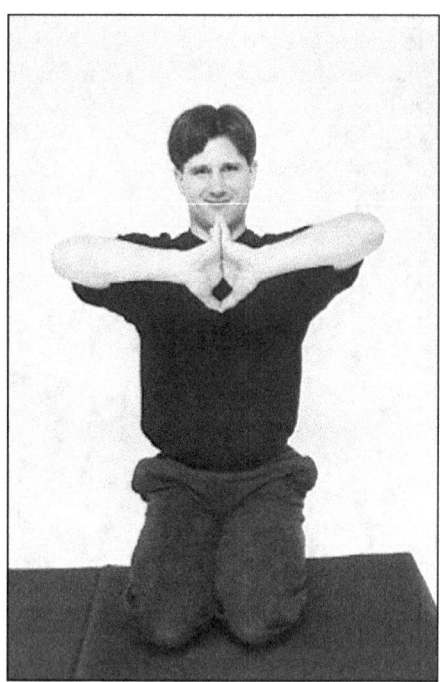

In this stretch you want to keep the area where your fingers join your hand (except for your thumb) together while pointing your fingers toward your chest and pushing out away from you. This affects the fingers, hands and wrists.

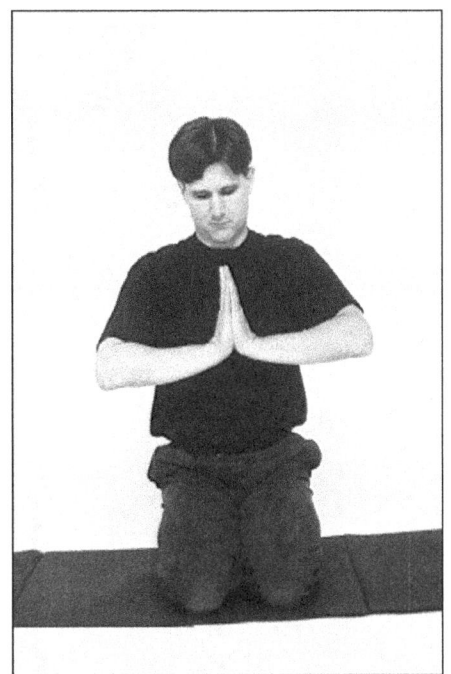

Keeping your palms together (where your hands meet your wrist) and your fingers pointing straight up, push your hands down toward your groin area. This stretch affects the carpal tunnel, wrist, and forearms.

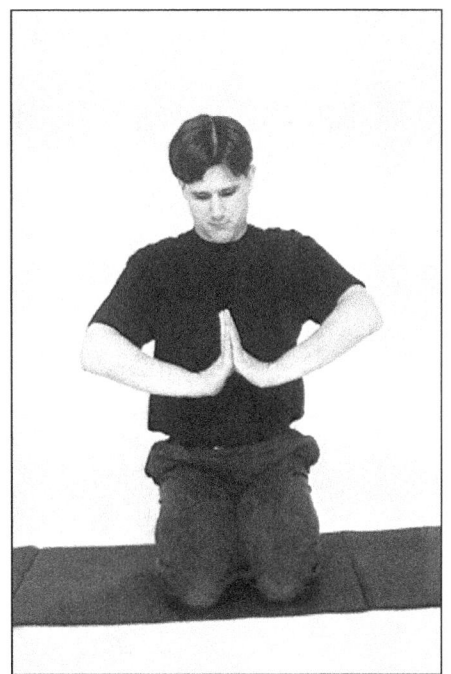

A variation of the previous stretch involves keeping the area where the fingers meet the hands (except for the thumbs) together while pointing the fingers straight up, opening the palms up, and pushing the hands downward.

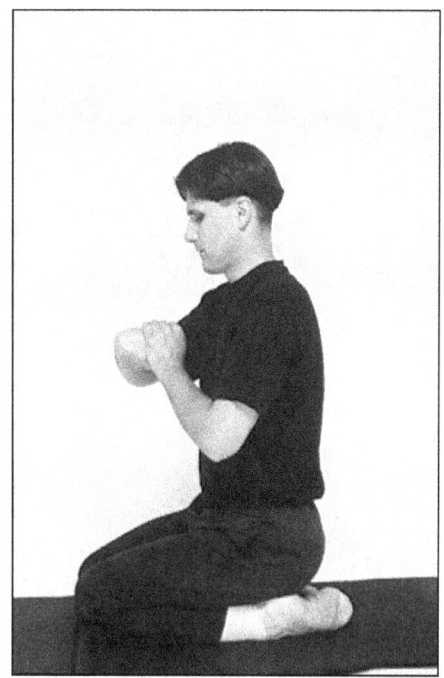

This is a great stretch for the outside of the hands and forearms. Make a fist with your right hand and point it in towards your chest at a 90° angle, using your left hand to keep it at a 90° angle while pushing outward.

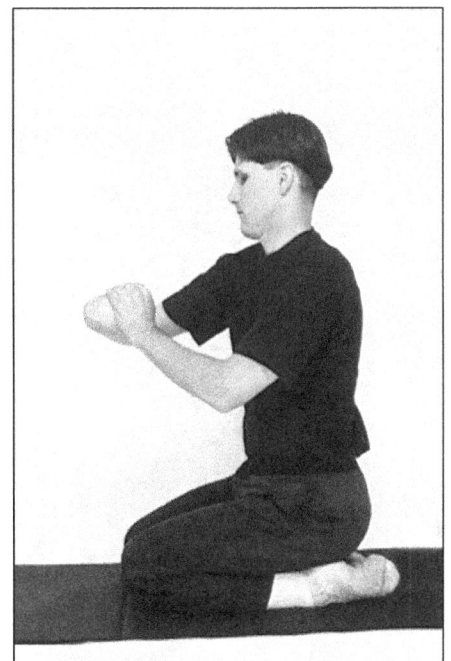

Continue pushing your right hand outward away from your body until the desired stretch is achieved. Be sure to stretch the left hand as well and always keep the hand at 90° to the body.

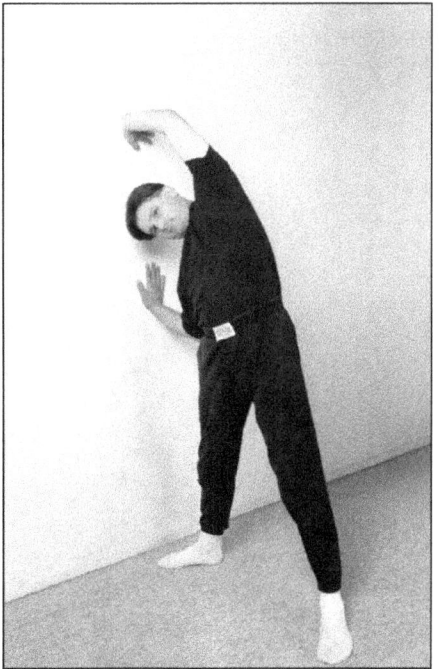

This **side stretch** is achieved by placing the left hand directly above the head while attempting to keep the body at a 90° angle to the wall and pushing away from the wall. Do the other side also.

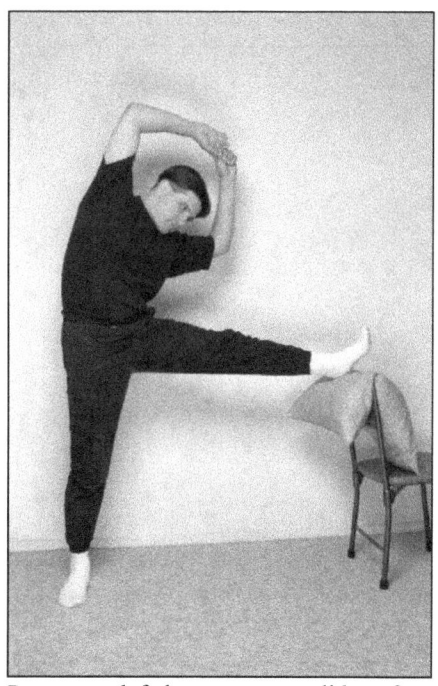

Prop your left leg up on a solid surface with your toes facing upward while using your left hand to pull your right arm over your head. Keep your left leg at a parallel angle to the floor. Do the other side too.

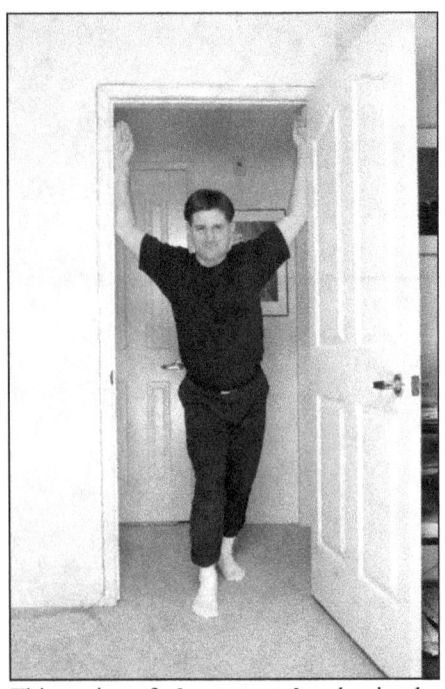

This series of **chest stretches** begins by placing your hands and inside forearms on a door frame and pushing your chest forward and away from the forearms and hands. Affected areas include the pectorals and chest.

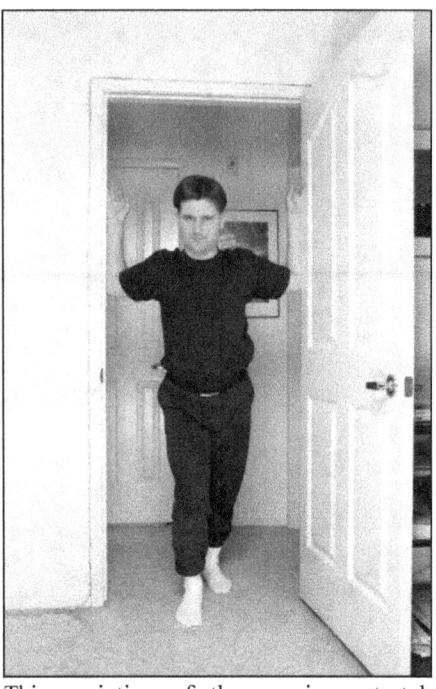

This variation of the previous stretch affects different muscles by placing your hands and inside forearms at various locations (up or down) on the door frame. Move the hands/forearms to the same area of the frame on both sides.

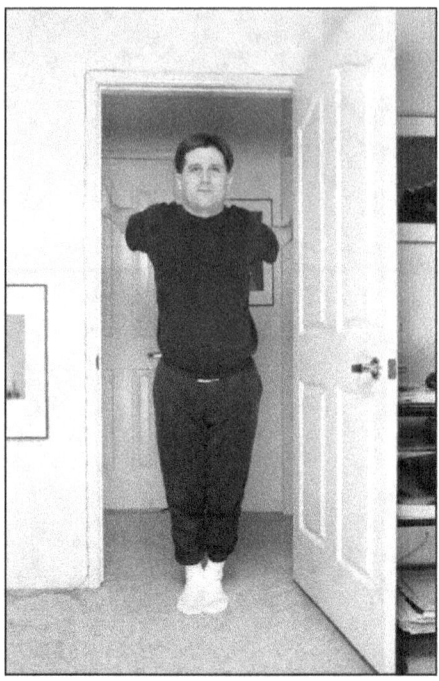

Place the palms of your hands on the inside of the door frame while moving your chest and body forward until your body is at a 90° angle to your arms. Move your hands up and down to various locations. This affects the pectoral/chest area as well as the shoulders.

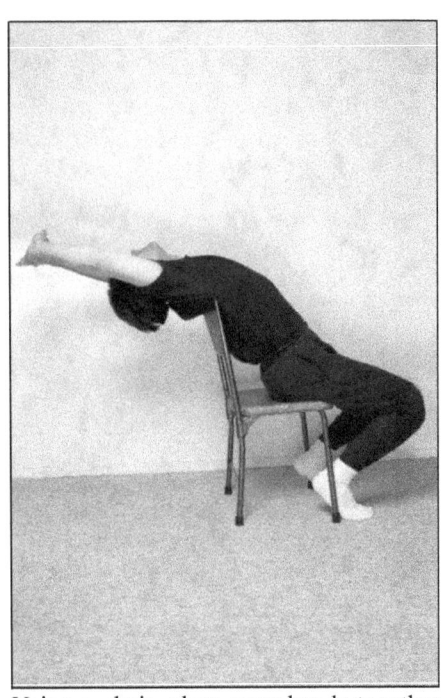

Using a chair, clasp your hands together as shown and lean backward on the chair while pushing your hands outward and down toward the floor. Bend your head back as well. Be careful not to fall backwards.

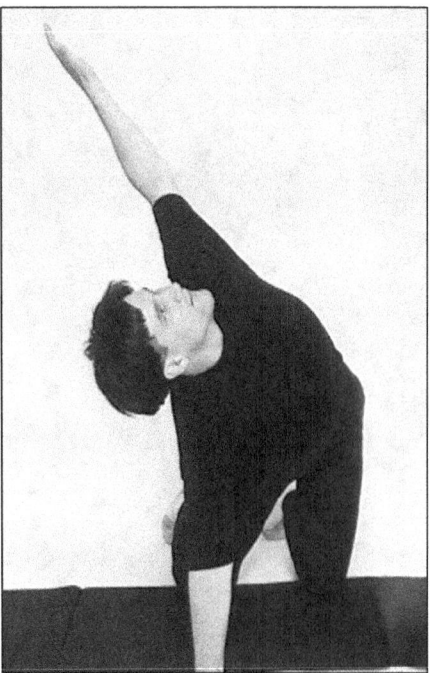

While keeping your arm straight, point your left hand toward the ceiling and the further behind you while keeping your right arm on the floor. Do the other side also. This stretch affects the chest, arms and back.

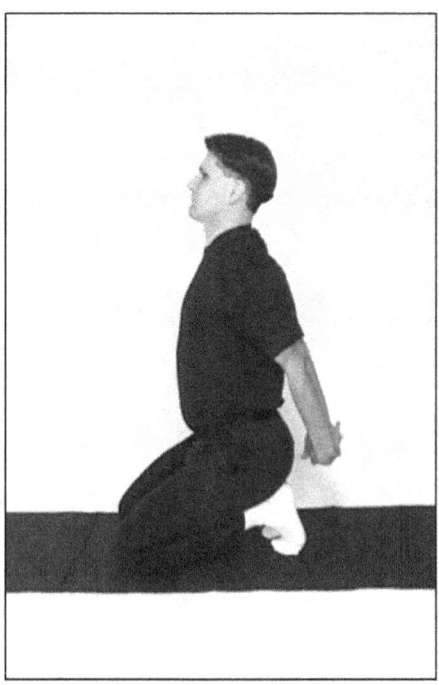

Clasping your hands together as shown, pull your shoulders back while keeping your back straight. You should feel a pull on your shoulders and pectorals/chest. This stretch is great for opening up the chest area.

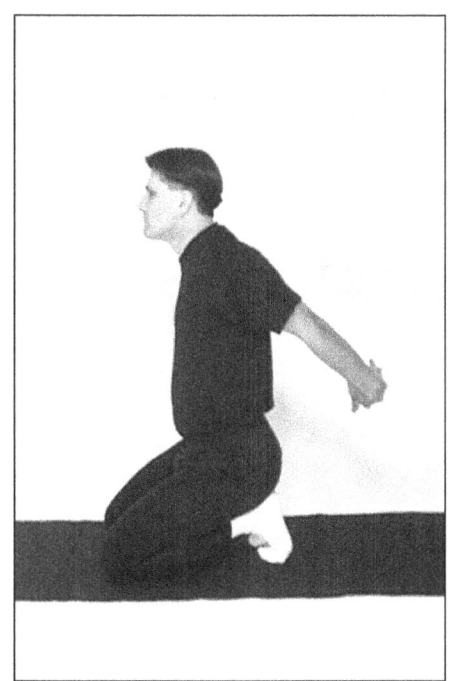

Using the previous stretch as a starting point, continue by slowly lifting your hands upward behind your back. Turn the bottoms of your arms in towards each other for a greater stretch. Lift your hands as high as is comfortable.

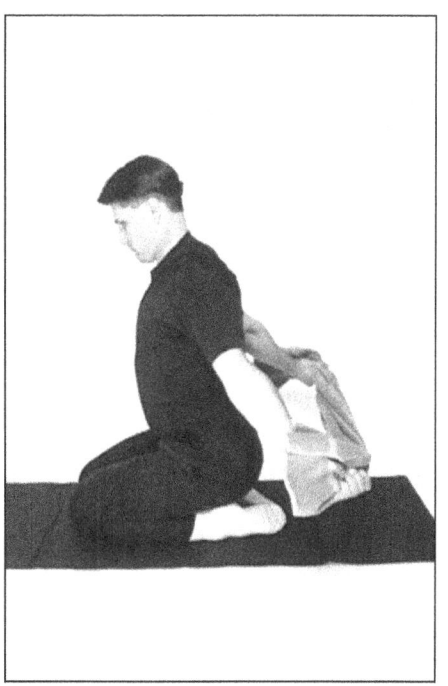

This is yet another variation of the previous chest stretches. Using a towel, grasp both ends with your hands as shown and slowly move your hands in towards each other until the desired stretch is achieved.

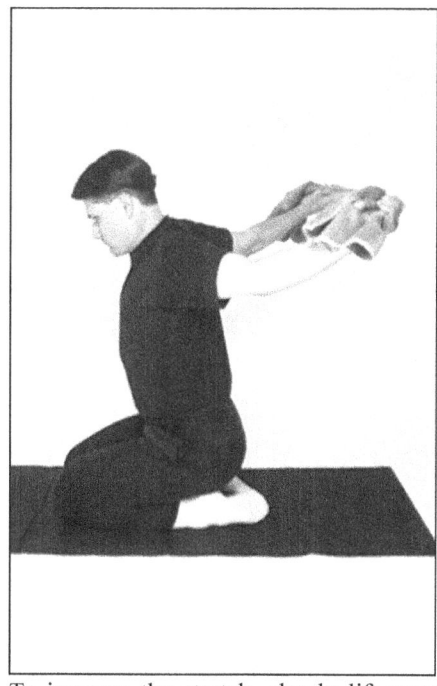

To increase the stretch, slowly lift your hands and arms up behind you until you find the desired stretch. Eventually you may be able to bring your hands and arms all the way up and over your head and in front of you.

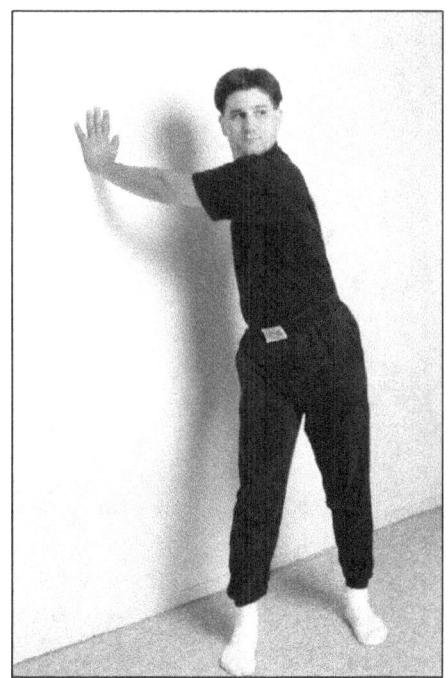

This **back and shoulder stretch** is great for the upper back and shoulder. Place your hands on the wall and move your left shoulder away from the wall. Turn your feet away from the wall and keep your left arm straight.

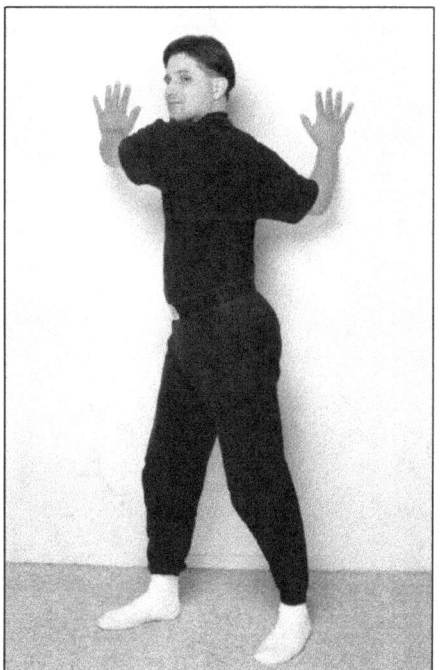

This is another view of the previous stretch. Increase this stretch by twisting your hips away from the wall, turning your head around, and looking behind your back. Be sure to do the other side also.

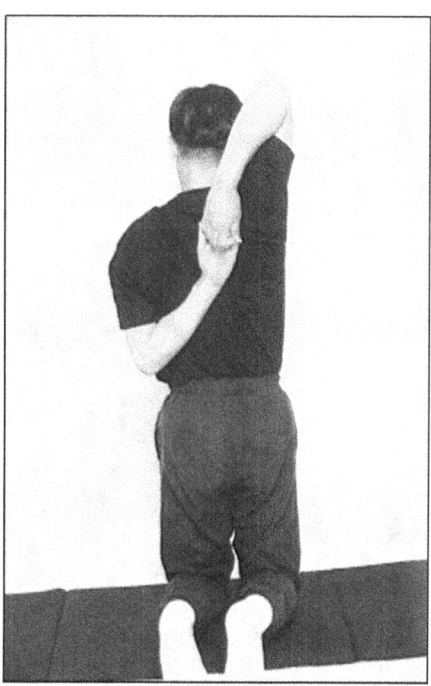

This stretch affects the left shoulder as well as the inside of the right arm. Clasp both hands together behind your back as shown. In time you may eventually be able to move your hands up your forearms. Do both sides.

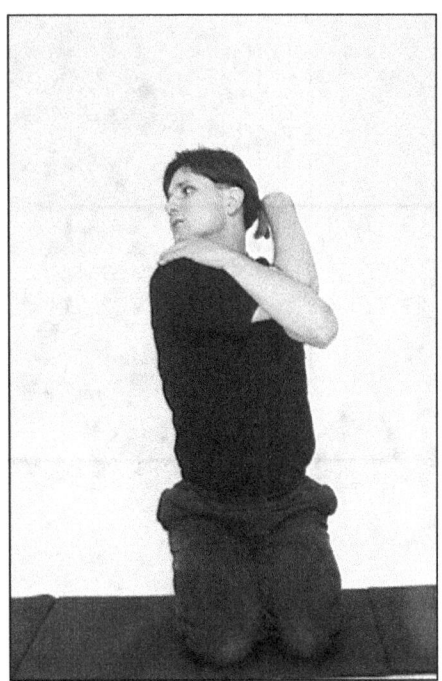

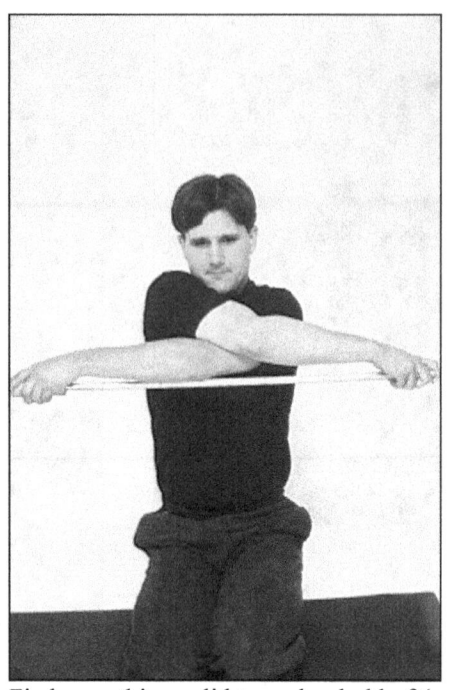

Place your right elbow into the joint connecting the fore and upper left arm and pull the right elbow to the left and up while applying downward pressure to the right shoulder with the left hand. Do both shoulders.

Find something solid to grab a hold of (a fence always works good for this stretch). Criss-cross your hands so that your arms are overlapping and slowly edge your hands out away from your body. This is great for the shoulders and back.

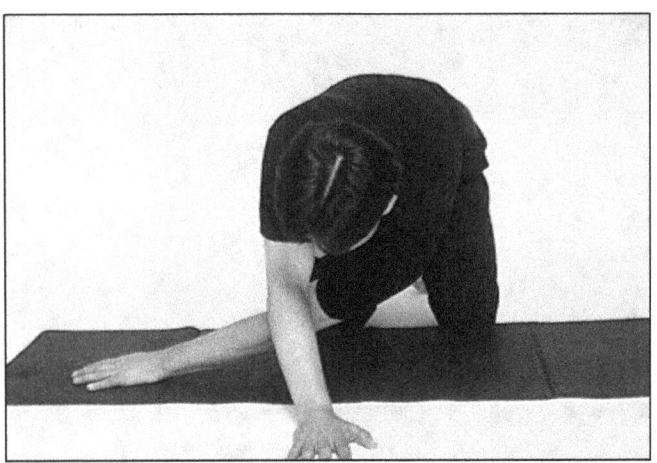

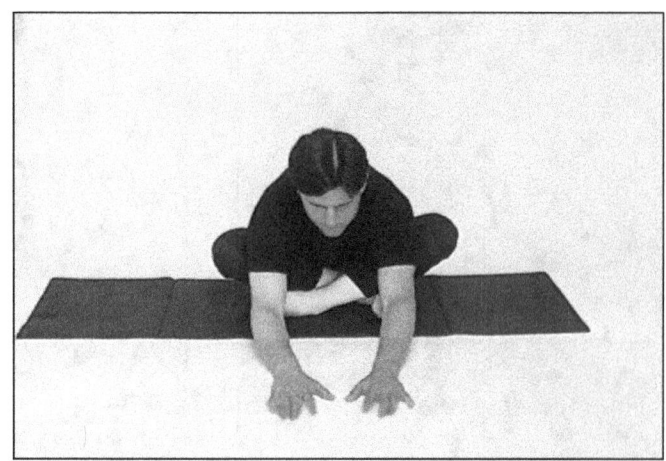

While down on all fours place your right hand out in front of you for balance while moving your left hand under your body and to the right on the floor. Continue nudging your left hand to the right until the desired stretch is attained. Do the other side.

To stretch out the lower and middle back as well as the buttock area, fold your legs up underneath you while leaning forward. Stretch your hands out in front of you as far as is comfortable. Be sure to bend from the lower half of your back.

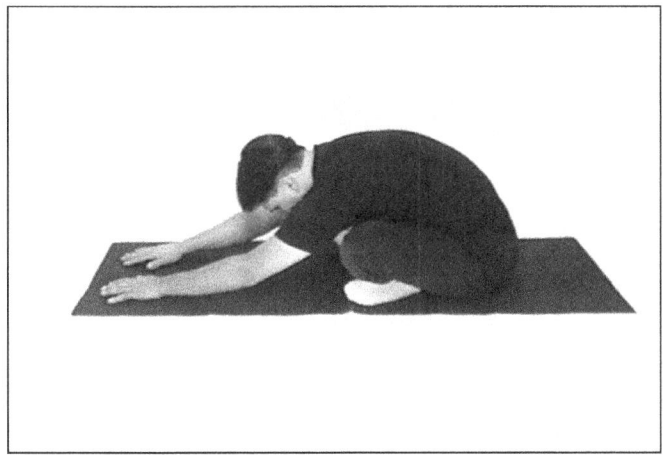

Here is another view of the previous stretch. Again, try to stretch from the lower back rather than the upper. Nudge your hands further away from your body to increase the stretch. Be sure to keep your buttocks on the floor.

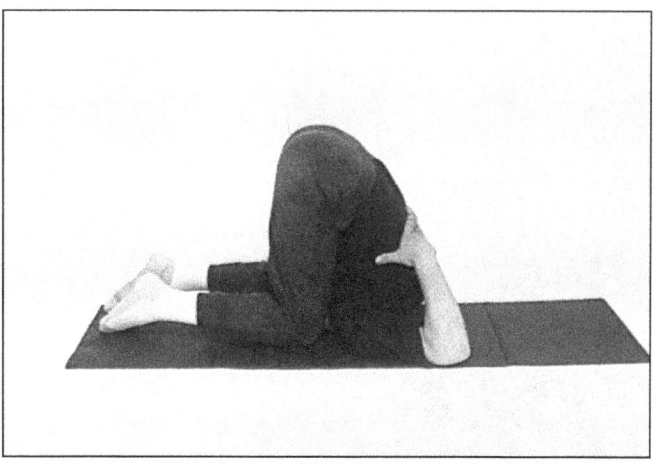

This is a great stretch that affects the entire back. Lie flat on the floor and throw your legs over your head, slowly lowering them until your knees are next to your ears and your lower legs are above your head.

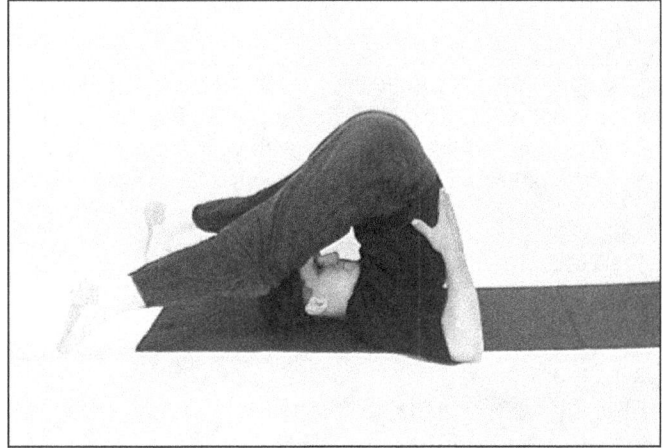

This is similar to the previous stretch and affects the upper and lower legs as well as the back. Start from the previous stretch and slowly extend your legs out above your head, being sure to keep your legs straight and apart. Rest on your toes.

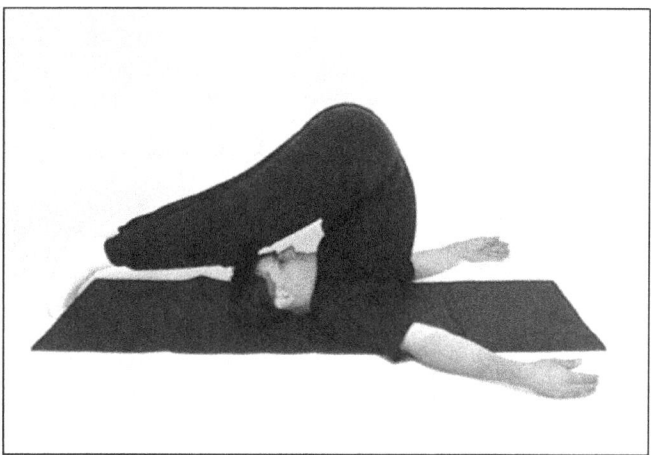

Start this stretch from the previous position by slowly moving your legs together while staying up on your toes. Then move your arms behind you. The main areas affected are the legs, buttocks, and lower back areas as well as the neck.

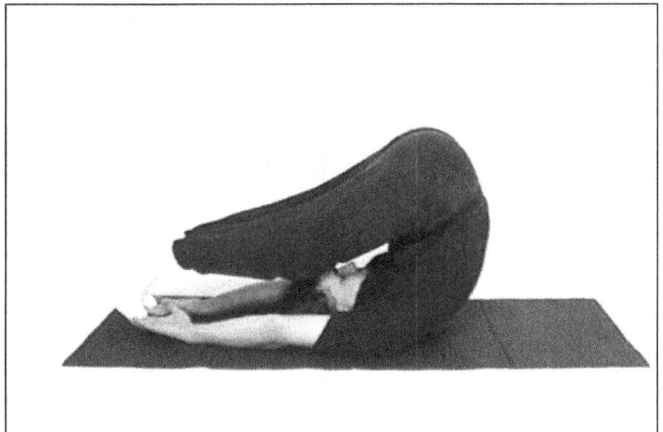

This stretch primarily affects the legs, buttocks, upper back and shoulder blade areas. Start from the previous position and then slowly bring your arms around to hold your toes. Keep your legs straight and together.

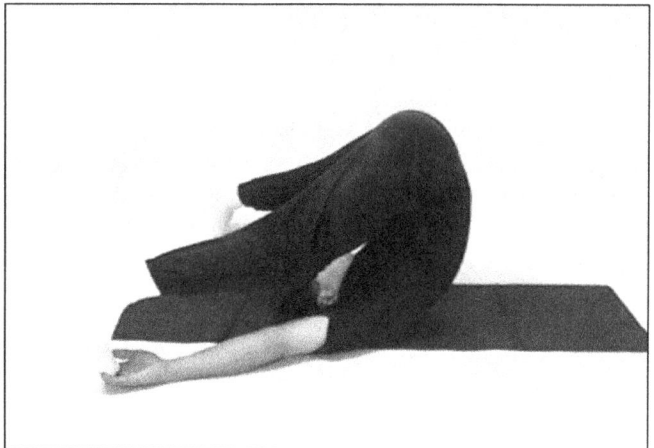

This stretch is a variation of the previous position and is achieved by starting from the former position and then spreading your legs apart while continuing to hold your toes and keep your legs straight.

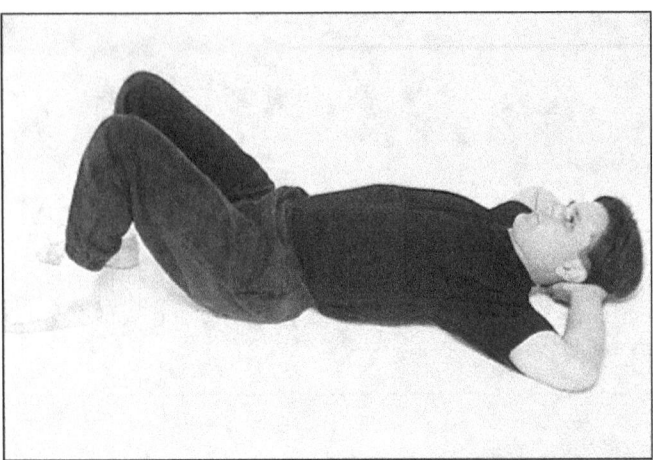

Begin this stretch by lying with your back on the floor. Proceed to lock your fingers together behind your head and pinch your shoulders together. This stretch affects the upper back as well as the chest and lat areas.

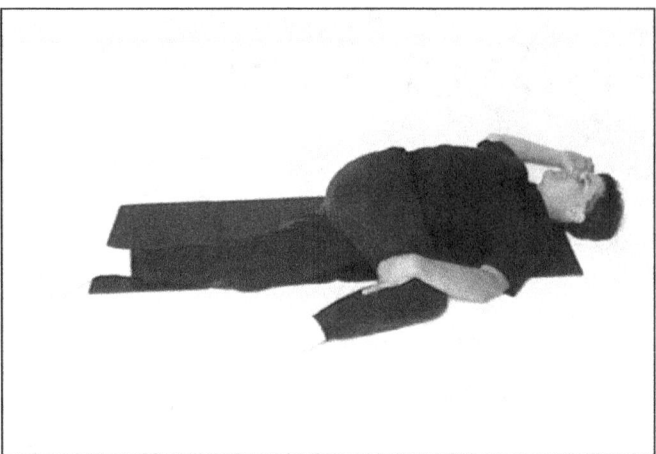

This is a great stretch for the lower back. Begin by lying with your back flat on the floor. Then raise your right knee up and pull it over your left leg to the floor with your left hand. Keep your right shoulder on the floor. Do the other leg as well.

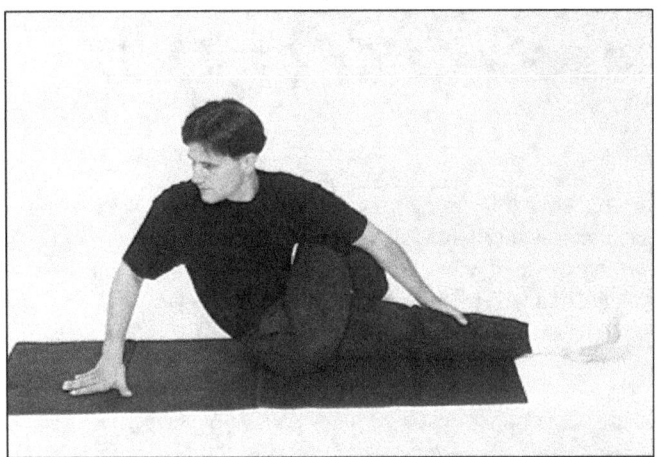

Sit on the floor with your legs straightened out in front of you. Raise you right knee up and place your right foot on the floor on the other side of your left leg. Place your left hand on your left leg and push your right knee away from you to the left with your left elbow. Turn your upper torso around to the right and looking behind you. Do the other side too.

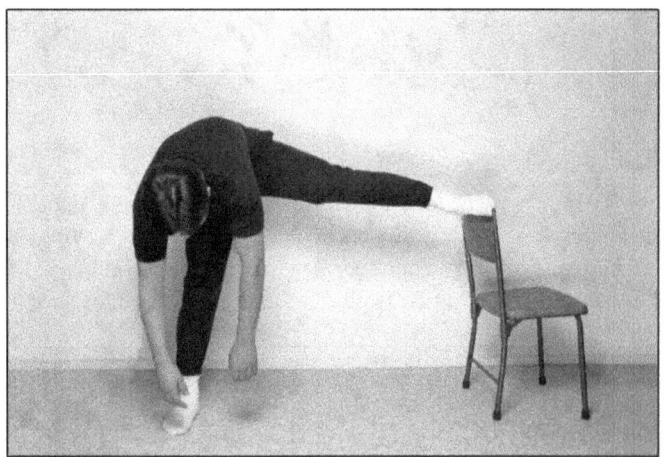

To produce this **leg stretch**, position your left foot on the top of the chair sideways and keep your right foot pointed straight out in front of you. While keeping your legs at a 90° angle to each other, bend your head and arms down, trying to touch the foot. Do the other leg as well.

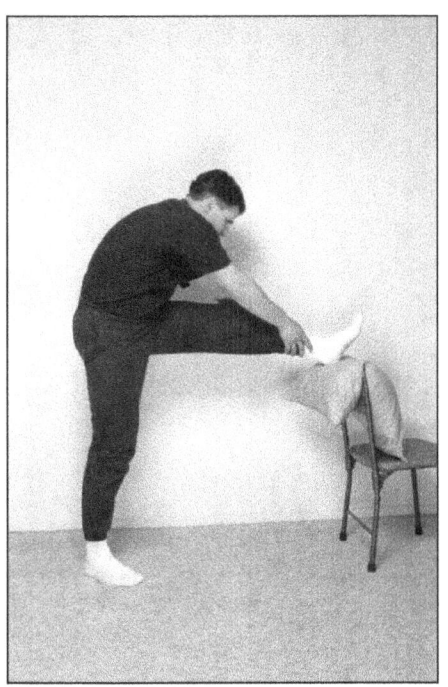 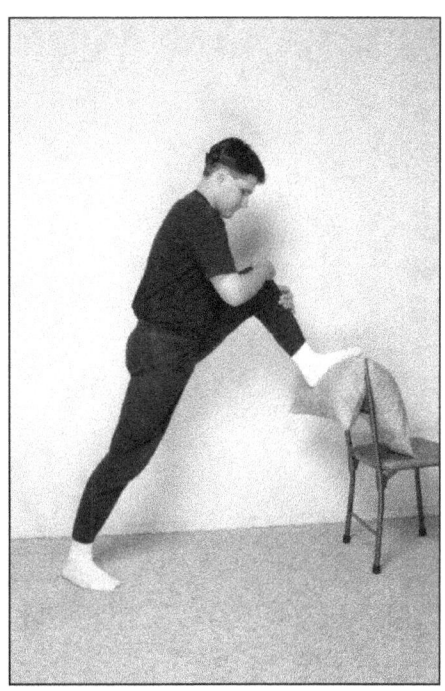 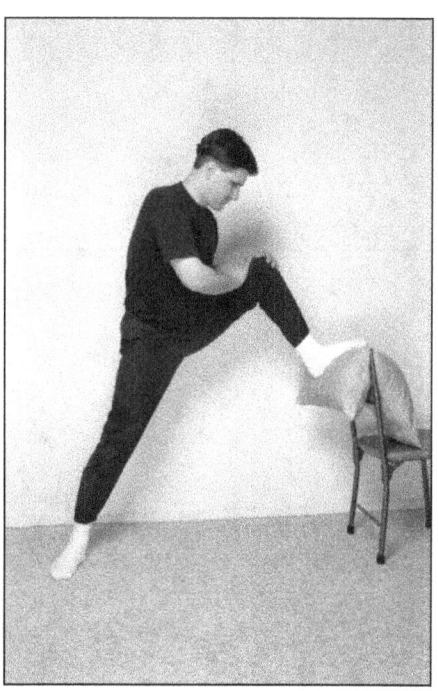

Another way to stretch the leg using a chair involves placing the left foot straight out in front of you on the top of the chair. While keeping both legs locked straight, reach forward with your upper body and grab your left ankle. Do the other leg also.

In this exercise, place the bottom of the left foot on the top of the chair while keeping the right leg facing forward. While keeping the right leg straight, bend the left knee and lean forward until a nice, easy stretch is felt at the ankle and upper leg areas. Do the right leg too.

This variation of the previous stretch is essentially the same with the exception that the straightened right leg is facing out (to the right) from the body. In both exercises you should try to lean forward from the hips. As always, do the other leg as well.

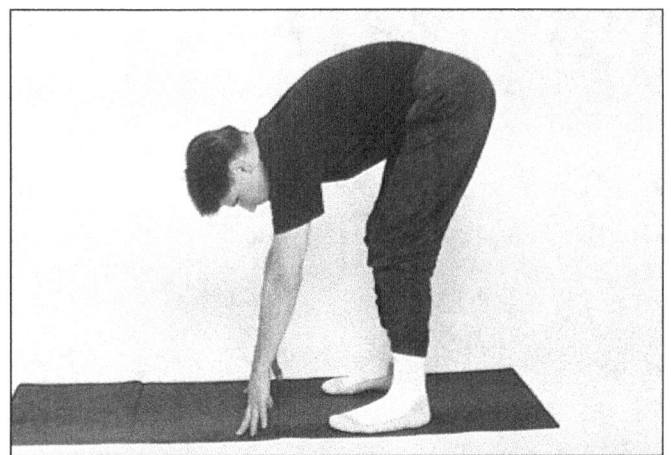 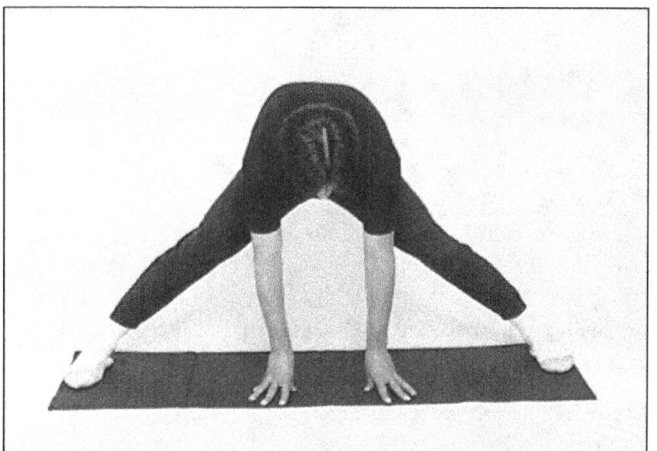

This exercise affects the entire back leg area. Place your feet about a foot apart from each other, and while keeping the legs fairly straight, bend down and touch the floor with your hands. Be sure the toes are pointed straight out ahead of you.

Place your feet apart from each other, being sure to point your toes straight ahead. While keeping your legs straight, lean down and touch the floor with your hands. You can obtain a better stretch by leaning from the lower back downwards.

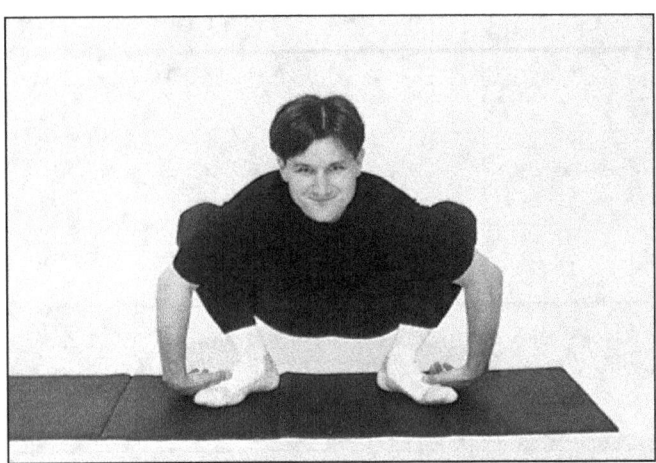

This stretch affects the inside upper thigh. Begin by squatting as shown from a standing position, supporting yourself with your feet (do not sit down). Then put your upper arms over (in front of) your knees and use them to push apart your legs.

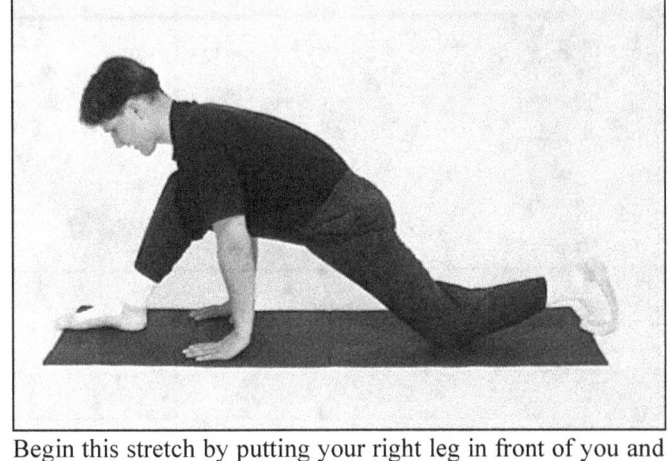

Begin this stretch by putting your right leg in front of you and your left leg in back of you. Scoot your right leg forward while pushing your groin toward the floor until an easy stretch is felt on the inside upper thigh of the right leg. Do the left leg too.

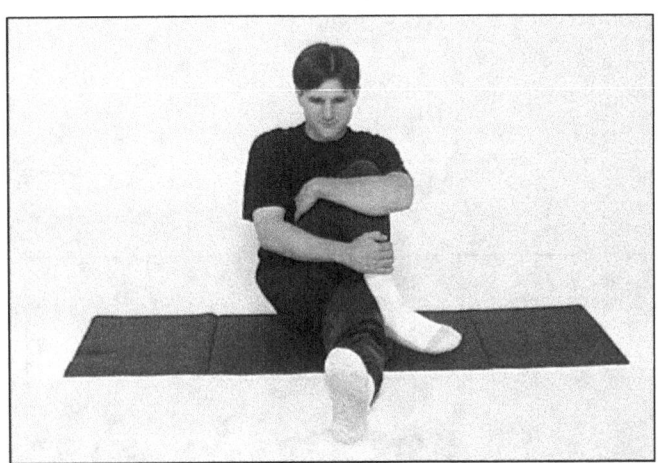

Begin this stretch by putting both legs in front of you. Then bend your right knee up and grab it with your left hand, pulling it over to the left. Finally, pull your knee into your chest with your hands and arms. Do the other leg. This stretch affects the buttock and outer thigh.

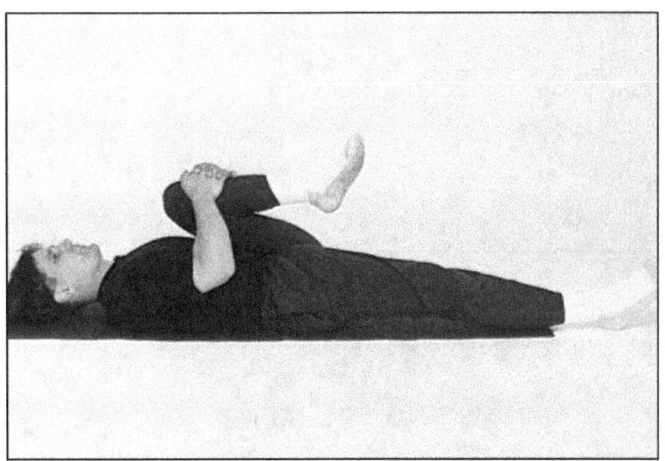

Stretch the upper back leg and outer buttocks with this stretch. Begin by lying on your back and raising your left leg up. Then grab your knee with both hands as shown and pull it into your chest. Do the right leg too.

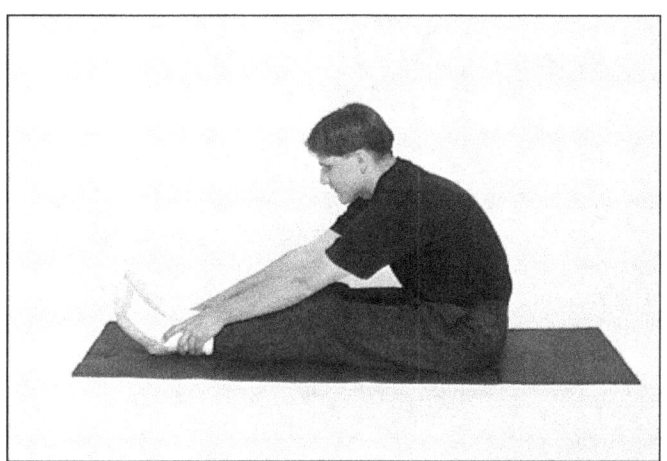

This exercise affects the entire back leg region. Begin by lying flat on the floor. Then sit upright and lean forward towards your toes, grabbing your ankles with your hands and slowly pulling forward until an easy stretch is felt on the back of the legs.

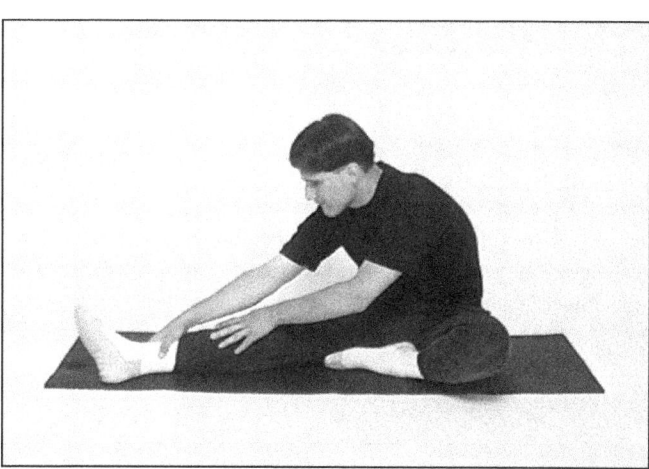

Stretch the back of the right leg by tucking your left foot up against your right inner leg as shown, keeping your right leg straight and your toes pointing up. Bend forward from the lower back towards your right foot. Do the left leg as well.

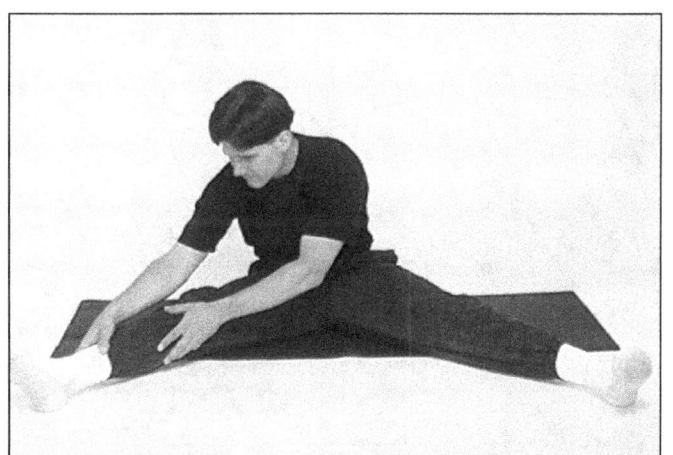

This variation of the previous stretch has the left leg being extended as well as the right leg. In this instance both legs are spread out and extended straight with toes pointed up. Lean from the lower back towards the right leg. Do the left leg next.

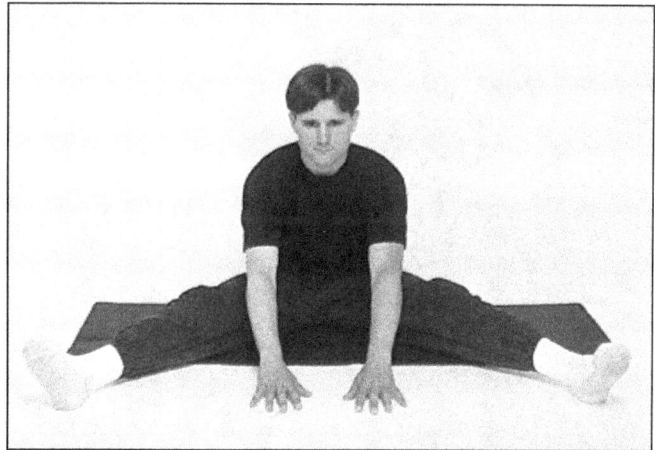

This is a variation of the previous variation, requiring the legs to be straight and the toes pointed up with this exception: in this instance you lean forward from your lower back directly in front of you. Great for the back and inside legs.

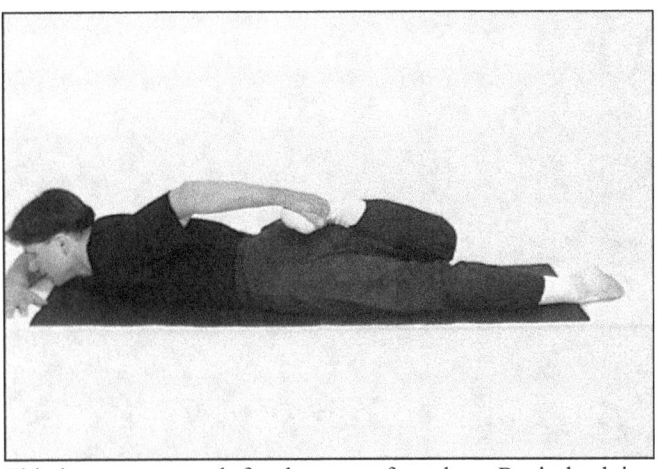

This is a great stretch for the upper front legs. Begin by lying face down on the floor; then reach behind you with your left hand and grab your right ankle/foot, pulling it upwards toward your lower back. Pull upwards more to increase the stretch. Do the left leg next.

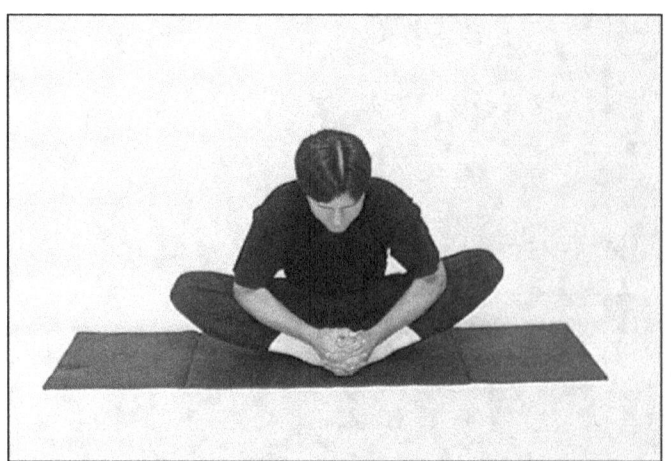

This stretch for the inner upper leg is achieved by sitting down on the floor. Put the bottoms of your feet together. Next, grab your toes and pull them in towards your groin. Use your elbows to spread your legs apart while leaning forward.

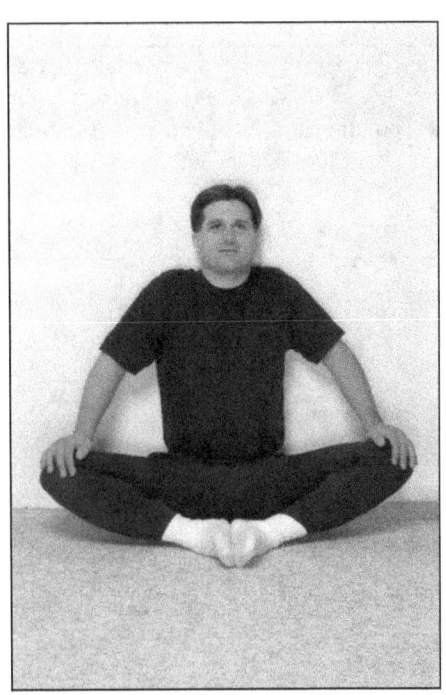

This variation of the previous stretch starts by sitting on the floor with your back against the wall. Put the bottoms of your feet together as before and pull the toes toward your groin but use your hands to push your knees to the floor while keeping your back against the wall.

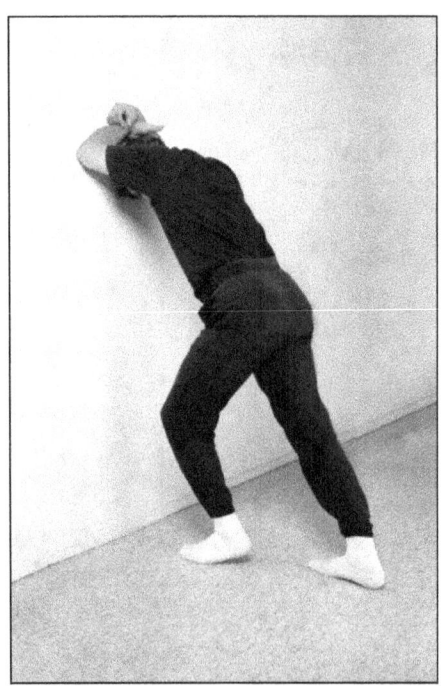

This series of **ankle stretches** begins by leaning on a wall with your forearms while extending your right leg behind you. Keep the toes of your right foot pointed straight towards the wall as you keep the entire foot flat on the floor. Do the left leg also.

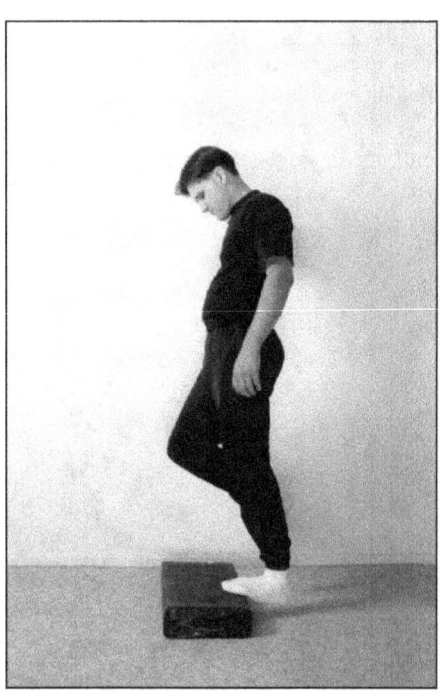

This ankle stretch is best done on a curb. Begin by putting the toes of the left foot on the edge of the curb using your arms (or your right foot) to stabilize your balance. Let the muscles of the left foot relax to get an easy stretch. Do the right ankle next.

Certain types of Yoga are also an excellent way to become more limber and are worth checking into.

EXERCISE

Exercise is a necessary part of any serious rehabilitative program. The right kind of exercise (aerobic) provides the oxygen required for tissue repair. In addition, aerobic exercise:

• helps loosen and tone muscles
• helps joint problems like arthritis by bringing oxygen into an area
• accelerates injury recovery
• helps the heart work more efficiently and prevents heart disease
• improves circulation
• enlarges and cleanses the body's capillaries (the small arteries that transport nutrients into muscle tissue)
• lowers blood pressure
• decreases hunger cravings so you eat less
• helps you lose weight by burning fat and calories (and continues to do so after the exercise has stopped)
• quickens the metabolism, causing the body's processes to work faster and more efficiently
• improves digestive elimination
• strengthens the immune system
• purifies the body of harmful elements
• increases high-density lipoprotein levels in the body (responsible for cholesterol management)
• relieves stress, depression and tension

The question isn't whether you should exercise or not but rather what kind of exercise is good for you and will not increase damage done. This chapter discusses the proper methods and techniques you must know to exercise correctly so you can create an exercise program that is right for you.

Some preliminary things should be mentioned. First, be aware that other daily activities that work injured tissue areas can compound problems already caused by playing or practicing and should be avoided. If you put in a lot of practice hours that cause elbow pain and then proceed to manually wax your car, the waxing is also taxing your elbow. You might believe your pain is caused solely by practice hours when in fact it could be a number of things unrelated to playing. Observe what you do during the course of the day that might have an affect on an injured area and make changes where necessary. This includes certain types of exercise so find exercises that don't over-affect the areas. This is especially true when beginning an exercise program for the first time.

Second, don't exercise heavily while fasting or going on a low nutrient diet. Heavy exercise demands higher mineral and vitamin amounts but dieting or fasting restricts the intake of these vitamins and minerals. This can cause light-headedness and other problems.

Third, stay warm when exercising. Training in cold weather should be avoided if possible. This is especially important the first few minutes you begin exercising. Remember to "warm up your engine" before you "drive off". Try to stay warm for the first five minutes of an exercise program. When you're at a job be sure to have a warm jacket and gloves for your hands if your are going to move heavy equipment in cold air (such as amplifiers).

I'd like to stress once more how important exercise is. Perhaps you've heard from different sources that you should immobilize the injured area and rest it. I have tried it more than once and it has been my experience that immobilization is the wrong choice. Think about it for a moment: after a period of time an immobilized area begins to weaken and atrophy. If you were to keep your arm in a sling for two weeks it would atrophy and weaken. If you were to then go out and use that arm (performing, perhaps), you would probably find (as I have) that the pain didn't go away and in fact may have gotten worse. This is because your arm is actually weaker than it was two weeks ago. You immediately went from "zero to sixty" when you took the sling off and performed. Rest is important but in most cases movement should be favored over no movement at all. Harmful wastes products also settle in injured areas if you don't keep your body in motion.

PROPER WAYS TO EXERCISE

Stronger people suffer less from overuse injuries. This is attributed to better endurance and the ability to withstand greater loads. For musicians, endurance is more important than the amount of load our muscles can bear. If properly set up, most instruments aren't really physically demanding until you've played them for many hours. Endurance becomes the issue at this point. If you were to practice two hours a day and then work a four-hour job you can easily see why endurance is important. Endurance can be attributed to two things: the strength of the individual and the aerobic fitness of the individual. Between the two, aerobic fitness is more important to endurance than strength when you speak of the amount of time muscles can go without exhaustion. Remember this: the more work you do, the more your muscle tissues need oxygen. Muscular endurance is needed through proper aerobic exercise.

Before beginning any aerobic exercise regimen be sure to maintain a diet high in complex carbohydrates to provide sustained energy levels. Do not eat before you exercise since your stomach requires blood from your system to digest food. This leaves very little blood in your tissues and joints, making them more susceptible to damage. Exercising before breakfast is usually the best time. There is a possibility of lactic acid build-up if you exercise later at night. It's also not a good idea to exercise when you're tired. Do your exercising in the morning when you're well rested. It will set the tone for the rest of the day: activity.

Establish regularity with your exercise program. Some people exercise every day; some exercise every other day. Many people say that your body needs a day off to recover from the exertion; I personally feel this applies mainly to weightlifting and not aerobic training. Whatever the case may be I would recommend an exercise schedule of no less than three days of aerobic exercise per week. Which schedule you choose is entirely up to you. Find a schedule that works for you and the amount of injury you are suffering from. Listen to your body and let it tell you what to do.

Above all, be consistent with your schedule. Maintain a regular exercise schedule. This doesn't mean exercising in pain. If your schedule seems to be causing you more pain, change your schedule or skip a day. At any rate, start off with an easy schedule. Begin your exercise routine slowly and make it progressively longer and more challenging over time. Don't overdo exercise. Moderate exercise is what's needed. A moderate workout combats stress and tension more effectively while an "addiction to a schedule" or heavy exercise program adds mental stress. Don't become an exercise addict. Learn to skip a day if you're in pain and don't start with a heavy training program. Besides, you can often maintain aerobic fitness by substituting one form of aerobic exercise for another. Switch from swimming to running for a few days if your arms hurt. Slow down if the injury doesn't seem to be recovering. It took you a long time to damage your muscles. It will take some time for them to recover. Relax. Over-training can result in injury, lactic acid build-up, disillusionment, and possible abandonment of your program.

Begin each workout with a mild body warm-up. This can be easy jumping jacks or running in place for two to five minutes. This oxygenates, warms, and loosens up muscles to prepare them for stretching. Do not skip this step as it helps prevent lactic acid deposits in tissues after exercising. After the initial warm-up, stretch your muscles according to the stretch routine that you designed for yourself, remembering not to be forceful. This prepares your muscles for aerobic exercise.

Begin the aerobic workout after warming up and stretching. There are many ways to work out aerobically and each way provides different benefits and problems. Some of the best are listed below:

• Walking is one of the safest and least damaging ways to get aerobic benefits. Be sure to go at a faster pace. It may also be a factor in the prevention of osteoporosis.

• Running is great as long as you have good running shoes and find softer surfaces to run on. The high impact nature of running can cause other problems but can be avoided if these precautions are addressed.

• Swimming is a great way to exercise aerobically and can build strength in the upper body. There is no impact involved as there is with running. Be sure to take it easy if you have arm or upper body problems. Go slow, there's no need to swim hard. I began by doing 2 laps a day really slow, fully stretching my arms while stroking. Avoid swimming in a pool for long periods of time as chlorine can destroy much of the body's vitamins.

• Dancing provides aerobic benefits. Additionally, being around other people can also improve your mood and take your mind off of your muscle problems.

• Bicycling is good exercise unless you have leg or wrist problems. Legs get quite a load put on them and wrists become very tense and stiff holding handlebars. It's a great way to exercise if you don't have these problems.

• Basketball is a tremendous aerobic workout if you become involved in a game. Find a local park and shoot a few or join a game. People with hand or wrist problems may suffer so try it out and see how you feel.

These are just a few good ways to exercise aerobically. You may find other ways to exercise that will also give you aerobic benefits. Experiment and find the exercise that's right for you that doesn't exacerbate the problem.

Spend at least half an hour on aerobic exercise, daily or otherwise. Be sure to inhale and exhale deeply while exercising as it helps get more oxygen in your system and carbon dioxide out. You should not be out of breath. You are pushing too hard if you have difficulty saying your name while exercising. Slow down and keep an even, regular, moderate pace. The energy and effort expended is not nearly as important as the duration. By the time you finish you should be perspiring slightly and feel your heart beating. During the last five minutes you should cool down slowly by going at a more leisurely pace. Conclude with some easy stretches. The last cool-down/stretch ritual assures a minimum of lactic acid and stiff muscles. This is the proper way to oxygenate your body.

There has been a controversy over the use of weights or handgrips with overuse injuries. While it's important to strengthen an area, it's good to keep in mind that muscles need to be limber in order to be quick. Whenever I have done hard physical labor I have found strong hands don't make for quick fingers. Furthermore, your muscles have probably spent the last few years tying themselves into tight knots if you have an overuse injury. The last thing you should do is tighten them more. After recovery you might want to rebuild strength in your recovered problem areas with weights to prevent future injuries. Stronger people do suffer less from overuse injuries. Weightlifting or handgrips at this point should be counterbalanced with stretching so muscles don't tighten up.

If you decide to lift weights be sure not to lift heavy weights. It is better to do many repetitions with smaller weight amounts than the other way around. Movement should also be unhurried and deliberate, covering the entire range that the limb can move. Divide your repetitions into two sets of ten repetitions each. Take a short break between repetitions. If the lifts become easier you can increase the weight amounts but be careful. This advice goes for handgrips or tennis/rubber ball squeezing also. My personal belief is that weightlifting, pushups, handgrips, or any other strength-building exercise should only be done after an injury is healed. It will probably take six months to a year before your muscles start to feel normal again so if you're beginning this program, don't even think about it. Stick with aerobic exercise only. In the beginning don't lift any heavy objects at all if possible. If you find yourself in pain again, stop. Focus on aerobic exercise rather than weight training.

CHAPTER 3: PLAYING HABITS

Most musicians don't think much about how they physically practice. We are too wrapped up with playing to stop and take a look at how we are playing. Musicians perform constant repetitive small muscle movements that increase the chance of an overuse injury. This is why overuse injuries are classified as repetitive motion injuries. Any serious rehabilitative program must take into account the lifestyle, habits or actions that caused the problem in the first place. And since greater and greater technique demands are continually expected of musicians, it becomes even more imperative that the issues of practicing and performing are addressed. This chapter discusses proper methods for practicing and performing, including mental attitudes. Use this section to evaluate your habits.

PRACTICING

It is unfortunate that ideas like **warming-up** or **stretching** before practicing are rarely discussed in schools or private lessons. With the increasing technical demands expected of musicians it is critical musicians think of themselves as athletes. You should make two to five minute warm-ups and stretching a mandatory precursor to practice time. Then start your practice time with easy exercises, gradually moving on to more difficult ones later. Just a few minutes before you start can make a huge difference in how you feel during and after practice. Be sure to take the time to do this.

Take a look at how your instrument is **set up**. Is the action unnecessarily high? Is it positioned in such a way that you have to make extreme or unnecessary movements to reach it? As an acoustic bassist I had older players telling me to set the action higher on my strings. There is no need to set string action high these days as amplifiers, pickups, and speakers allow volume to be increased while action is lowered. The acoustic bassists I have met possessing great facility have their action set where it is as low as possible without compromising tone. Indeed, it would be virtually impossible to be able to play many things with high action.

Be aware of the **relationship of your instrument to your body**. For example, it makes more sense to have the neck up high close to your face on electric bass so your wrist is straight. Some people play with the neck of the bass hanging down near their belt area. Instances such as this cause the performer to bend their wrist in an awkward position to be able to play the notes on the neck. Needless to say, this can cause problems in the future. Question how you are holding your instrument and how it sits in relation to you, even if this goes against the traditionally taught methods. Make changes that make logical sense and feel right for you. Always make the job of playing an instrument easier when possible.

Your **posture** affects how you feel afterwards. Bad posture can affect how blood gets to different areas in your body and may impede oxygenation. Your shoulders shouldn't be slumped forward but pulled back and aligned with your chest. Keep your back straight. You may find that accessories used by other instrumentalists may work well on your instrument and may help your posture. I find that a classical guitar footstool helps me maintain good posture on electric and acoustic basses and relieves the need for me to use a strap on electric bass. This takes pressure off my neck and shoulders. You might even try more conventional solutions like an orthopedic stool. There are also many straps available today that aid in weight distribution of an instrument. I use the "Slider" dual shoulder strap. To me it just doesn't make sense anymore to play with a typical strap that puts all the weight on one side. Save yourself some future pain and get one of these.

Are you taking long, deep inhalations and exhalations when you **breathe**? Observe your reactions when approaching a difficult section in a piece of music you've been practicing. Do you breathe in short spurts or do you hold your breath? If either of these apply it's a sign of muscular and mental tension.

Your **frame of mind** regarding mental stress and hang-ups about music you are performing can cause muscle tension, which in turn can cause mistakes. These mistakes can cause further mental stress, creating a vicious cycle. Try this: think about playing a difficult section of music you are working on without actually playing it. What is your body doing? Are you tensing up? Your first response is to attack the mental problem by believing you can perform the section successfully. Envision being in a relaxed state while the notes flow out of your fingers effortlessly. Your mind has considerable control over your body. Think about the way your muscles feel when you are resting in bed and apply that feeling to playing. Then pick up your instrument and be consciously aware of your muscles as you practice. Zone in on them and use your mind and mental imaging to relax them if they are tense. It's common for musicians to expend more energy than required and tense-up when playing a difficult section. Relax and don't be stiff. Re-train yourself to be relaxed, loose and flexible while playing.

Awareness of the **sound** produced while playing your instrument provides a type of biofeedback if you listen to your tone when you play. Is the sound tense or forced? Don't just focus on technique or the physical playing of the instrument. Notice the end result of the sound you produce and actually <u>hear</u> what you are playing. Finally, come back to your breathing, being sure to take long deep breaths through the nose to assure maximum oxygenation. These concepts help relieve muscle tension which tires you quicker, causes your muscles to remain tense permanently by knotting up (unless you stretch the knots out), and is a major contributing factor to overuse injuries.

The amount of **time** spent practicing affects how you feel as well. Your problems will get worse if you maintain a frame of mind that your body is a machine you have complete control over. Musicians are notorious for spending extraordinarily long hours practicing. The concepts in this book will extend your endurance but you must realize the body can only take so much. If you are suffering from an overuse injury the best way to start practicing again is to divide your practice sessions into small amounts, taking small breaks in-between. Begin with 15-minute practice sessions separated with 5-minute breaks where you stand up and stretch your muscles. You can eventually increase practice sessions to 20 minutes, 30, etc. all the way to an hour as you begin feeling better. Shorten your practice sessions to less than 15 minutes if 15-minute practice sessions cause pain. The key is to play without pain by listening to your body. Don't increase practice time unless you are sure you are playing without pain. Always stretch between practice sessions.

Most importantly, **don't practice if you hurt!** You will occasionally push too hard and re-injure yourself as you learn to adapt to your new habits. Forget about your regiment or schedule at times like these. It's O.K. to skip a day if you need to. Take as much time off as necessary to return to normal and try to identify what you did to re-injure yourself. The time off will also clear your head of stress and tension, allowing clear introspection to help solve musical problems you were working on. Sometimes thinking about a problem with a stress-free mental state away from your instrument allows a solution to present itself.

PERFORMING

Practically all ideas pertaining to practicing apply to performing also. There are two main differences between practicing and performing:

- People are listening to you when you perform
- You can't stop playing to go back and fix a problem when you perform

These two differences create other problems including a fear of making mistakes, a fear of being judged for mistakes, and a new and unfamiliar environment that can lead to distraction and a lack of focus. All these issues add mental and physical stress and tension. Dealing with these issues in a positive way is a major factor in any successful performance and contributes to how our muscles feel during and after performance.

Start applying your **practice habits** to the performance. Warm-up and stretch before a performance, be sure your instrument is adjusted correctly, check your posture, listen to your tone, etc. Initially it will be difficult to think about all these things while performing. They will eventually become unconscious habits if you spend time now to think about them while performing.

Be sure you **know the material to be performed**. I often see musicians stumbling through a piece because they didn't spend enough time to completely learn what they were going to perform. This frazzles a performer's nerves, adding stress and tension to the mind and body. It's much easier to completely know the material so you can perform calmly, relaxed, and confidently. You will personally enjoy the performance more if you are not worrying if your technique will be sufficient to play a passage or whether you will forget certain parts. Adequate preparation lowers stress levels.

Think about what you **eat and drink** before and after a performance. Alcohol should be avoided as it affects how your muscles react as well as your brain's response time. Coffee, soft drinks and tea all contain caffeine that may cause a jittery feeling in your muscles. Personally, coffee causes me to play slightly faster and rush. It's preferable to leave these stimulants out of the work environment. Sugar or sugar-containing products are not recommended as they may make you slightly hyper and are bad for your muscles.

The **amount of food** eaten prior to a performance also has consequences. Eating just a little bit of food can combat any nervous butterflies you might feel on an empty stomach. On the other hand, eating too much food makes you tired as your system attempts to digest it, leading to a poor performance. Over-consumption of food also causes much of the blood in your system to go to your stomach for digestion, leaving little blood in muscle and joint tissue. This has an affect on how your muscles feel afterwards. Since blood brings nutrients in and waste products out of muscle tissues it is not recommended to put this kind of stress on your muscles during peak performance times.

Finally, **forget about what your listeners think.** You want them to enjoy themselves of course but it's a waste of time to worry about their reactions. Their reactions are out of your control. The only person you have control over is you so just be yourself and enjoy the moment. Whatever insecurities you might have about an audience's negative reaction to your performance are probably unfounded anyway. Don't worry about it. It's difficult enough to perform without worrying about what your listeners think of you. Concentrate on the job at hand. It has been my experience that if the band is having fun the listeners will pick up on that energy and have fun as well (whether or not they actually understand the music). What kind of energy are you sending out?

CHAPTER 4: REST

Musicians have difficulty getting adequate rest since many keep irregular hours doing club work or touring. Sufficient rest must be achieved if one is to recover from overuse injuries. Your body uses sleep hours to make repairs to your body, including muscular tissue. Adequate amounts of sleep at regular intervals are critical for this reason. You should get at least **seven hours of sleep** at night if possible. This is especially important if a regular sleep schedule is not maintained.

Establish a regular **sleep schedule**. Regular, consistent hours help the body repair itself quicker and more efficiently. Go to bed at the same time and wake up at the same time. Your body has an internal clock that needs to be set to run efficiently. When your body's internal clock is set it has found what is called a "circadian rhythm". It takes a couple of weeks for your body to set a circadian rhythm so it is important to keep regular hours.

Your sleeping arrangements affect your sleep patterns and how efficiently your body repair's itself. Lumpy, soft or saggy mattresses affect body alignment and cause muscle pain as a result. Consider what can be improved. I have found a futon mattress laid directly on the floor to be the best thing for muscular problems. There are other kinds of special mattresses as well: mattresses with magnets in them, mattresses made of special materials, orthopedic beds, etc. You might also want to check out orthopedic pillows. It will take some experimentation to improve your sleeping arrangements.

Finally, take two consecutive days off a week where you do nothing but relax. Give your muscles a rest. Most people work five days a week and take the weekends off. A musician's life should be the same. Breaks are necessary recuperative time.

CHAPTER 5:
PSYCHOLOGICAL STATE
ATTITUDE

I recall wondering if I'd ever get over my injuries. I was repeatedly told that once a person has tendonitis they'll always have it. I began to believe this after all the doctors, chiropractors, acupuncturists, and others had unsuccessfully tried to relieve me of pain. As a result I developed a very dark attitude. I wrote this section to encourage you to **never give up**. I know how frustrating it can be. I've been there. You have to keep your attitude together.

Consider how much your thought affects how your body reacts. Do you remember how you felt on your first date? You were probably nervous with butterflies in your stomach. Your perceived **mental** issues with acceptance (i.e., "do they like me?") caused a **physical** change in your body. Your heart beat faster, your stomach was nauseous, and you might have been sweating. These physical symptoms originated from a thought. Imagine how your body might respond if you feel pain every time you pick up your instrument. After a number of years it might become conditioned to associate playing an instrument with pain and begin developing physical reactions to just the idea of playing an instrument. If you expect to feel pain when you play it is very possible the increased mental stress and tension surrounding playing is causing physical responses (such as tighter muscles). Your thoughts may even create the physical pain itself in anticipation of playing! This is an obvious impediment to your recovery. For this reason you must **believe with conviction that you will recover from your injuries.** Beliefs that overuse injuries never heal don't promote recovery and can actually thwart it from happening. Maintain a confident attitude about your recovery. Changing your attitude toward your situation can be one of the most powerful tools in your recovery program. Re-consider your attitude and keep a positive frame of mind. I got over my injuries; I believe you can too.

When you find a treatment or program that seems to make you feel better, **use it to give you hope** to continue. A treatment that makes a difference can be powerfully reinforcing. It can change your attitude toward your situation and make you want to find more treatments that help. It also helps you gain control over how you feel. This is the real issue. The most frustrating part of having an overuse injury is the sense you are not in control. You feel like a helpless victim of the injury. Finding a treatment or method that works teaches you how to control and alleviate the pain. Knowing you are in control of how you feel can tremendously improve your mental state, which can improve your physical state. Use successful treatment methods as a tool to return to a positive way of thinking.

Your **social life** can affect your attitude. Mulling over your problems alone at home isn't good and can be harmful since you remain focused on the problem. It creates additional mental stress and physical changes. Get out of the house and distract yourself from problems. Visiting friends can be positive as it can lift your spirits and cause you to focus on other issues in a conversation. Good friends also provide emotional support that can give you a renewed sense of hope about your situation. You may even find your problems are not so big in comparison to a friend's. Get out of the house and enjoy yourself.

Finally, why are you playing music? What is your motivation? Are you competing? Why did you originally pursue a career in music? Most people decide to become musicians because they love playing music. This is the best reason to practice and perform. **Play music because you love it.** Musicians are often in a comparison mode of thinking and compete as a result of it. This kind of thinking makes you feel you are wasting valuable practice time and falling behind other musicians when you slow down to take care of injuries. It also makes it difficult to appreciate accomplishments you've made since you may feel self-acknowledgment of your talent might cause you to become comfortable, relax, and slow down. This all stems from a perfectionist type of attitude, which creates enormous amounts of stress. Don't torture yourself. Acknowledge and enjoy your accomplishments. What's the point in playing if you can't enjoy the strides you make?

CHAPTER 6:
TRAVELING

The road presents multiple problems for those who want to try these ideas. Rest and diet are not always in our control when touring. Time zone changes give you jet lag. Still, there are things you can do to minimize the effects of the road on your changed lifestyle patterns. Here are some examples:

• **Set your watch to the time zone of the place you're going to** before leaving. This way you can begin adapting to it while in transit or even before you begin traveling. Adjusting your sleeping and eating patterns earlier can minimize the effects of a time zone change when you arrive.

• Understand that **sunlight helps your body find a sleep schedule**. When you arrive in a country in a completely different time zone it is wise to stay up and go outside during the day (even if you are tired) so your body can adapt quicker to the new time zone. Walking outside in sunshine helps your body realize it's daytime and begin finding a circadian rhythm. Staying in your room will make it harder for your body to adapt and take longer.

• Remember that **a big meal can make you tired**. Don't eat a big meal if you are having difficulty staying up during the day. Eat just enough to hold you over until evening.

• **You have control over the food available to you**. There are many instances where you can be creative and find healthy food choices. You might go to the salad bar, get some vegetables, and make a salad dressing of half oil, half vinegar, mustard, and pepper. Easily obtainable healthy vegetables at a salad bar include celery, romaine lettuce, spinach, tomatoes and onions. This conforms to the "no refined foods diet" and actually tastes good. Think creatively for ways you can eat healthy when traveling.

• **Take a short nap** if you absolutely cannot stay up. 30 minutes is usually enough to revive most people a little. Sleeping more than an hour may make you feel groggy or affect your ability to sleep later in the evening. Put an alarm clock at the far end of your room so you have to get out of bed to shut it off. Ask for a wake-up call at the front desk also.

• **Don't exercise late in the evening**. The energy from exercising will make it difficult for you to get to sleep. It is also not advisable to have a big dinner before retiring. Eating a big dinner (especially with refined carbohydrates) less than 3 to 4 hours before bed can create a tremendous amount of energy that must be worked of or it gets converted to fat or acid.

• **The time you get to bed** depends on when your performance is over. I generally try to get to bed at around 11 or 12 if possible. Use your best judgment based on your circumstances.

• **Set the T.V. in your room to a channel with static** if you are having trouble sleeping due to inconsiderate neighbors or other sounds. Turn down the volume just enough so you don't hear the external noise. The steady hum of static can drown out the other sounds and lull you to sleep.

These tips help lower stress on your mind and body, lessen the effects of jet lag, and can reduce an overall worn-out feeling. All traveling situations differ so it may not be possible or practical to completely adhere to these ideas. Incorporate as many as you can and use your best judgment based on your situation.

CHAPTER 7: TREATMENTS

This section covers possible treatments for overuse injury problems. It is the culmination of nine years searching for remedies for my ailments of tendonitis, bone spurs, and carpal tunnel syndrome. I have included all remedies I know as well as some I haven't tried since I learned of them after I recovered. I have also included the remedies I consider to be bad ideas. **These remedies are to be tried in addition to good nutrition, supplements, stretching and exercise**, not as a substitute for them. At the very least you should be taking vitamins A, B, C (with bioflavonoids), and E, should not eat refined foods, and should stretch and get aerobic exercise. This is the <u>minimum</u> required if you are to get better. Try some of the other supplements listed in the "Supplements" chapter to see if they help. Actually, they all help. The limiting factor is how many supplements you want to take and how much money you want to spend. Then try some of these remedies for a week at a time to see if they make a difference. If they do, add them to your arsenal to combat your injuries. The concept is to keep trying new treatments, adding the ones that help to your recovery program so the combined effective treatments will speed recovery and give you renewed confidence in your program.

I have purposely refrained from recommending one particular method of dealing with overuse injuries for everyone (other than the minimum listed above). There are two reasons for this. First, we are all genetically different and may respond to various treatments differently. Treatments that work for me may not work for you. Second, the way you injured yourself may be different from the way I injured myself and therefore your body may not respond favorably to treatments that worked for me. Who we are genetically and how we got our injuries can make all the difference in how our bodies respond to a treatment. <u>You</u> have to do the investigative work to find the ones that work for you. These treatments are listed so you know they exist and can try them.

I would like to re-state that I have listed all the treatments I know of, including ones I don't recommend. I included these in the event you may be considering them and try to give advice based on what others have told me after undergoing the treatment. I believe it's a good idea for you to be aware of all alternatives and treatments available. If I don't think a treatment is a good idea I will tell you as well as give my opinion on treatments I have tried. There may also be effective treatments that have recently come out that I am not aware of so you may want to try them as long as they seem safe. Use your best judgment.

Acupressure is one of the oldest healing arts in history. The fact that it has been around so long is a testament to its effectiveness. Ineffective treatments don't last long. Acupressure is based on the idea that your body has certain areas called "pressure points" that can stimulate blood flow and healing responses in damaged areas when violated. This violation consists of finger or elbow pressure of a certain amount applied to the pressure points. Two other similar methods to acupressure are Myotherapy (which combines stretching with violations of greater intensity) and Rolfing (which is deep tissue massage that incorporates violations stronger than Myotherapy). All three methods can dramatically help the healing process. They may be painful at times but they unquestionably stimulate blood flow and break up scar tissue. I have walked out of

Myotherapy appointments where my body seemed like it was on fire because of the amount of circulation going on. It is a very warm feeling and I can't recommend these methods highly enough.

If you can't afford treatments or don't have anyone to work on you it is possible to use a tennis ball as an acupressure tool for back problems. Lie down on the floor and put the ball between the floor and your back, finding spots that seem to be a problem. Lean into the ball, apply pressure for about a minute; then release. It's important to apply the right amount of pressure. Too much pressure may aggravate muscles more while too little may not be helpful. Learn the right amount through trial and error and try various angles when you press. Try using a tennis ball in a hot tub or sauna also. You may find a connection between one area of the body and another by pressing at different spots; I found that pain in the knuckle on my middle finger was directly related to an area on my arm 2 inches above the wrist. Experiment.

Acupuncture is an ancient healing art that is often recommended for overuse injures. The concept of violating the body to stimulate blood flow is similar to acupressure. Both acupressure's and acupuncture's goals are to reset your "chi"-the energy channels that flow through the body. According to this philosophy, muscular aches and pains result from improper "chi" flow where the "chi" is blocked up. Some believe "chi" is the electricity that flows through your body while others maintain "chi" can be observed through Kirlian photography (the photography that shows the aura of a limb even after it is severed-"Phantom Limb" Syndrome). My personal experience has been that acupuncture did not have lasting results. Some of my friends have claimed it helped them considerably. If you don't mind needles you might want to try it for a little while to see how you respond.

Anti-inflammatory drugs such as Advil or Motrin may temporarily relieve pain but do nothing to solve the underlying problem in my opinion. In addition, prolonged use causes ulcers and some experts believe they may break down joint structures. I constantly needed to take more Motrin to get the same pain relief. As it is with other drugs your system becomes accustomed to the drug and eventually requires more of it to get the same effect. I started out taking 500 mg. of Motrin at a time and was at 2000 mg. at a time when I quit. It is not a solution. A much safer solution for temporary pain relief is bromelain pills. These are completely natural anti-inflammatory pills made from pineapples that don't cause the aforementioned problems. Juicing fresh pineapple stalks (where bromelain is concentrated) is even better. Anti-oxidant supplements also help reduce inflammation and assist in tissue repair. Topical solutions (such as Tiger Balm) are good for temporary pain relief.

Anti-oxidant supplements reduce inflammation and promote permanent healing. Free radicals are harmful substances in your body that cause inflammation. Anti-oxidants combat free radicals. Any substance that helps your body retain more oxygen for longer periods of time promotes tissue repair. Oxygen is the key to tissue repair and anti-oxidant supplements help your body retain oxygen. The supplements listed in Chapter 1 provide maximum oxygen-retaining benefits for the body. There are plenty of other great anti-oxidant supplements as well. Do some research and try different ones to observe the effect they have on you. This is only limited by your time and the amount of money you want to spend.

Adding **apple cider vinegar** to your diet has been purported to dissolve the calcium deposits responsible for arthritis and bone spurs. People use apple cider vinegar to clean calcium deposits left on the sides of a coffee pot so it theoretically makes sense. Calcium deposits and bone spurs are typically formed by the body as a way of adding extra strength to a heavily used joint. The body may go overboard, however, creating excessive deposits that can grate against muscles and nerve endings. It is thought that apple cider vinegar only breaks down the excess deposits while leaving the actual bone calcium alone. This is because excess deposits are not part of the bone matrix and are separated from bones by a protein coating. I have had bone spurs but not arthritis and would say that apple cider vinegar treatments should last for a long period for it to be effective. Use caution as it has also been reported that too much may result in the bone itself being broken down. Try a cup filled with half water and half vinegar for a week to start off. You might also try making salad dressings with apple cider vinegar.

Here is some advice I received from medical professionals regarding arthritis. You should avoid citrus fruits and especially orange juice. They are very acidic and may aggravate your joints. Vitamin C is necessary but take a vitamin C supplement that delivers vitamin C in a less acidic form (like "Ester-C"). Be sure they contain bioflavonoids as well. Taking a lot of oils (particularly fish oils like cod liver oil) can reduce pain and improve flexibility. The pain reduction is due to anti-inflammatory properties in fish oils. Vitamin E is another anti-inflammatory that is especially effective for coping with arthritis pain. Arthritic joints are "dried out" (they have basically rusted and oxidized) so oils are helpful and provide ease of movement. Finally, avoid over-ingesting animal fats, eggs, and dairy products. These have been shown to cause inflammation with arthritis.

Calcium is recommended for muscle aches. I have found calcium works great. You should take it with magnesium so it is utilized better. There are many calcium/magnesium supplements on the market.

"Chi" is not only a description of your body's energy flow but also a technique to relieve neck stress. It is harmless and can be performed in this manner: take one hand and put it just below your ribcage, putting your thumb on one side of your stomach muscles and your forefingers on the other side; then take your other hand and position your thumb and forefingers in the same fashion just above your pelvic bone. Lightly squeeze and press gently downward, holding this position for about a minute. Do this while lying down. I have had varying degrees of success with this treatment for neck tension.

Chlorophyll works so well that I wanted to list it here again for emphasis. Be sure to buy the "DeSouza" brand since processing methods vary. I have had no effect with other brands. Get three 1-pint bottles and drink one full bottle a day for three days. You may want to wait until you feel substantial pain to more clearly notice the effects. The first time I tried this method my pain was gone within half an hour. Truly amazing stuff! If you achieve similar results it probably means your body chemistry is screwed up. The relief you feel from the chlorophyll is the result of it equalizing your body's PH balance. This indicates your diet is affecting how you're feeling. Make changes.

Colon cleansing therapies are a good idea as body toxins often reside in the digestive tract. Many products are wonderful for cleaning you out. The best ones I've found contain psyllium husk. Removing toxic waste products should be a priority as they can often cause seemingly unrelated problems. Do colon therapies before a fasting program so you get the maximum benefit from the fast. A clean colon also helps in the absorption of nutrients. Colon cleansing is only necessary once a month as maintenance if you have a good diet.

Cortisone is not recommended and should be avoided unless all other options have been used. Your body produces cortisone and artificial cortisone tends to shut down the natural cortisone in your body. It may disrupt certain body processes. I have never taken a cortisone shot. Many doctors refrain from using it as a treatment. It is not as bad as surgery but would be my last choice before surgery. In all fairness I should say that some musicians have told me cortisone shots helped them. Others have told me it made things worse in the long run. Try other things in this book for a year or two before considering it.

Cracking and popping joints is a method many chiropractors use and can be helpful in relieving pain and tension. It helps re-align your body, opening up pinched muscle areas and increasing circulation and blood flow to the nerves. The sound itself comes from synovial fluid that rushes into a hollow area quickly. It should be mentioned that too much cracking and popping can cause arthritis (your joints begin to get a build-up of calcium deposits) and therefore should not be overdone. The most effective chiropractors I've seen do relatively little cracking and instead focus on other things like vibration, massage and stretching. Incidentally, if you tend to crack and pop a lot it is typically a sign of a bad diet, lack of rest, or inflexibility.

DMSO (Dimethyl sulfoxide) is used by athletes and sports medicine therapists. It's a plant derivative that is applied topically and promotes circulation to an area. It also makes you itch. DMSO acts as a transporter, carrying things directly through the skin into the bloodstream. You might try using DMSO with cod liver oil to increase the amount of oil absorbed through the skin. Be sure to wash your hands and the areas you want to apply DMSO thoroughly before use as it will carry whatever was on your skin into your blood as well.

Electric shock pulsing devices are used by chiropractors and are effective in relieving muscular pain and tension as well as promoting circulation and stimulating nerves. Two pads are placed on opposite ends of a muscle or muscle group; then electric shock pulses cause the muscles to contract and release, independent of your control. Unfortunately, these devices are difficult to find in the United States. Japan is one of the countries I know of that sells them. I own an Omron Vivi Elepuls HV-FO2. It's a small electric shock pulsing device that fits in the palm of your hand and costs about $50 to $100. Omron is a Japanese company that manufactures many health related devices including personal ultra-sound devices. Pick one up if you can get them. These devices feel good and seem to help. Be aware of the power setting as they can be quite powerful. Caution is advised.

Epsom salt baths help draw toxins through the skin and out of your body by osmosis. It also helps reduce swelling. Don't make the bath too hot. Remember that heat can cause engorgement of the tissues. Pleasantly warm is all that is needed unless this is your once-a-month toxin cleansing hot bath. If you live near an ocean an even better choice might be spending time in the salt water. The ocean contains lots of other minerals. Soak for about an hour. I have found this very helpful.

Fasting detoxifies the body and can contribute to overall health. It may cause queasiness as your body rids itself of the garbage it has accumulated over the years. In a sense, it's almost as if your body re-suffers through all your previous illnesses as it uncovers them one at a time. This has never happened to me but some of my friends have suffered these effects. Since fasting can be somewhat taxing on the body it is not recommended to fast frequently. Once in a long while (perhaps bi- yearly) is sufficient.

A particularly helpful type of fast is the lemon juice fast. Combine three cups of freshly squeezed lemon juice with a gallon of distilled water, fasting for three days while drinking a gallon a day of this mixture. Lemons are used since they are the only natural food that is anonic while water is catonic. This mixture of these two gives you a perfect PH balance, which enables cells to normalize and promotes rapid healing within the body. Every cell in the body has positive and negative ions, acids and alkalines. Think of the cells in your body as car batteries; drinking lemon juice and water is similar to adding more acid and water to a low car battery. In effect, it gives your system a "boost". Too little acid or water can cause problems in a car battery; this is why the <u>amount</u> of lemon juice to distilled water is important. Too much lemon juice can be very acidic and detrimental to healing. I have found this type of fasting to be helpful.

Ginger thins out the blood, reducing congestion that causes muscular aches and pains. Other purported benefits are headache relief as well as relieving nausea. I personally haven't found any significant change in my system by taking ginger.

Heat is not good for overuse injuries. Heat brings blood into an area (which is good) but it also increases inflammation and swelling. Heat causes the dilatation and engorgement of capillaries and tissues by bringing an overflow of blood, creating more pressure and potentially adding to existing damage. A damaged area is already inflamed by the injury. You don't want to bring more blood into an inflamed area already congested with scar tissue, crystallized lactic acid, and other waste products. The problems caused by heat are compounded further if your diet includes dairy or high sodium foods. The ideal situation is to bring blood into the area while simultaneously causing the inflammation of the capillaries and tissues to go down. Ice is therefore recommended. Heat is one of the best things you can do for yourself after an injury is healed, however.

Hydrogen peroxide or oxygen therapies make sense in theory. The concept is to ingest highly oxygenated liquids or hydrogen peroxide (the safe, ingestible kind of hydrogen peroxide-**do not drink the household cleaning type**) in an effort to increase the oxygen content in your body. Theoretically this increase in oxygen should speed recovery of overuse injuries. These special oxygenated liquids can be purchased at health food stores and are expensive. If you decide to try this be sure to do colon therapy first (clean out your colon) as well as drink cranberry juice to clean out the body's filters and waste channels. Then follow the directions on the label. A purported effect of this kind of therapy is experiencing prior illnesses as your body flushes the remnants of them and cleans you out. It made no noticeable difference in how I felt.

Ice is wonderful for overuse injuries. It stimulates blood flow to an area (the reason an iced area turns red) while simultaneously decreases inflammation and swelling. The blood flow brings needed oxygen to the blood vessels in the area. Use ice on an area whenever you feel pain or after a practice session or performance. My routine was going to the gym and soaking my arms and hands in a cold dip for 15 minutes. I would fill the ice bucket in my hotel room and pour the ice into the bathroom sink with some water if I was on the road.

Don't force yourself if you can't make your target ice submersion time. Listen to your body and use discretion. It's possible to cause nerve damage by icing an area too long but it's highly unlikely as the pain would be so excruciating you would have to pull out.

Kombucha mushroom tea has been purported to help overuse injury problems. It's a tea made from a giant mushroom and is an old Chinese remedy. I have tried it for common muscular aches but not for tendonitis and can't say for sure whether it helps or not. Friends have reported temporary beneficial results. There are probably many beneficial nutrients in the tea so I would recommend trying it to see how it affects you. These mushrooms can be hard to find but are often bought at health food stores.

Magnetology is the study of how magnets affect the body. Each cell in your body has positive and negative ions. The theory behind magnetology is that circulation can be increased by applying magnets to different affected areas, due to the movement of the cell's ions in relation to the magnet's polarity. There are many magnet products on the market to try: sleeping mattresses filled with magnets, magnet balls to roll around in your hands, magnet patches to stick on the surface of the affected area, etc. Some people swear by it. Rolling magnet balls around in my hand seemed to help me. These items are available at health food stores.

Manganese-containing supplements make the body's ligaments and cartilage more pliant. Supplements like Ligaplex 2 and Mag-Cal (which also contains calcium) are great healing agents that help in tissue rejuvenation and repair. Unfortunately they are also expensive. The same benefits might be provided by a high vitamin and mineral diet and Knox unflavored gelatin. Incidentally, gelatin is made from the tendons and hoofs of animals (horses). You must replace damaged tissues with tissues that are most similar to the damaged tissues (gelatin).

Massaging and vibrating are non-damaging methods designed to increase blood flow in damaged areas and are highly recommended. The increased circulation in an area speeds the removal of waste products and brings nutrients in. Massage and/or vibrating works out knots caused from overuse as well as ganglion tendons caused by atrophy that impede circulation. They also help remove scar tissue and lactic acid from injured areas. These are great ways to feel good and speed your recovery. Ask a significant other to give you a massage. You can also schedule an appointment with a licensed masseuse. Full body massages can really help make you loose. As for vibration there are several good massage vibrators on the market. I use a foot massager with a thick soft foam cushion over it. Be sure to put a foam cushion between you and the vibrator so you don't exacerbate your injuries. Be aware that too much time spent using a vibrator can aggravate an area. A half hour should be sufficient. Massage vibrators can be bought at reasonable prices and are wonderful for your muscles.

Niacin increases blood flow to an area by causing dilatation of blood vessels. It's found in the B complex. Over-ingestion of niacin is not recommended as it could possibly cause engorgement of tissues in damaged areas. Use in moderation and follow directions on the bottle. You should notice your hands turning red, your body feeling warm, and an itchy sensation when taking niacin; this is a normal effect. Niacin pills should be thought of as a temporary measure to help your body heal. The smaller amounts of niacin found in a B complex supplement are fine for daily use.

Oil used with a heating pad relieves pain, increases flexibility, and promotes healing. The process is this: pour a small amount of cod liver oil into a dishwashing glove. Tape the end of the glove shut with scotch tape so the oil doesn't leak out. Then wrap/tie a heating pad (set at a medium temperature) around your hand securely and sleep with it on. It is, of course, <u>never</u> recommended to sleep with a heating pad on so I cannot advise you to do this or recommend it.

This treatment had an amazing effect on my carpal tunnel syndrome. My pain was gone the next day. Cod liver oil is the recommended choice for oils as it contains high amounts of vitamin A and beta-carotenes. It's arachidonic acid, the lightest oil your system can break oil down to. One might say it has a very light viscosity if we use the car analogy. The lighter the viscosity, the easier the flow of the oil is. The cod liver oil essentially bypasses your digestive system when you put it in a glove. The use of a heating pad opens up pores in your skin, allowing the oil to be absorbed directly through your skin and into your muscle tissues. Like a rusty car door, the oil helps prevent "rusting" and "squeaking" (aging) and promotes flexibility.

An interesting thing happened when I attempted to re-use the glove used the night before. I was surprised the next evening when I found that the previously used glove had expanded to about one and a half times it's normal size. The oil saturated the glove and it became flexible and expanded. It occurred to me that this might also be what happens to my muscles.

Other things I tried with the glove treatment were hydrogen peroxide (the safe kind), carrot juice, orange juice, wheat germ oil, chlorophyll, and cod liver oil with DMSO. The hands must be very clean before doing these treatments as other things on the skin surface may also be absorbed. This treatment may be applied to other areas of the body through the use of cellophane and scotch tape instead of a glove.

Opening up the ileocecal valve unblocks food and waste products congested in the intestines. The ileocecal valve is located between the large and small intestines. Food occasionally causes other problems in the body when it gets jammed up in this area. To open up the valve, do this:

• Find the ileocecal valve-it's located on the right side of your body, midway between the highest part of your hipbone and your belly button. It's at a 45% angle between the two places.

• Lie down, take your left hand, position it at this spot, and use your fingers to **gently** push in and pull up towards your left shoulder. You are doing it wrong if you feel any pulsation beneath your fingers. You want to get beneath the valve and push it up. Lifting your right leg may help.

The valve often gets clogged up when you eat too much or too fast.

Reflexology is primarily concerned with how the body's systems and structures are interrelated and interconnected. An example of its use might be lightly tapping around the knee of an overuse-injury affected arm to help relieve tennis elbow in that arm. Lactic acid often accumulates at nerve endings in body areas that are connected to other parts of the body. The extremities often have nerve endings that are connected to other places all over the body. Tapping or applying pressure to these nerve ending points often results in increased blood flow to an area and dispersal of lactic acid crystals present. This results in pain relief at the interconnected area. I can personally attest to its effectiveness.

Rubbing the carpal tunnel is a great way to break up scar tissue and crystallized lactic acid. To do this, find your carpal tunnel (about the center of your wrist on the palm side of your hand where the muscles/tendons go through) and rub up and down over the tunnel. This rubbing should be lengthwise (i.e., toward your fingertips, then back towards your arm) and should not be painful. Just rub it enough to break up the scar tissue/lactic acid. Don't press too hard or you may hurt yourself. I found this to be very helpful. I remember feeling things breaking up in the tunnel the first time I did this. Follow this up with wrist stretches.

Saunas or hot baths are good when done once a month. They help get rid of toxins that accumulate in your body. The toxins are expelled through your skin by sweating. Vitamins, minerals, oils, and other important nutrients are also expelled, unfortunately. For this reason you should not take a sauna or hot bath more than once a month. Daily visits to the sauna or hot bath may cause you to lose the important nutrients your body needs to heal.

Spirulina is more effective for your mental state than your physical state. I mention it since your mental state can affect your physical state. Spirulina is an algae with a very high vitamin B12 content. B12 injections are often given to manic-depressive patients at medical hospitals. It can help your mental state and depression (particularly if your diet isn't good). It relieves depressed mental states and lowers stress levels. An effective tool for improving emotional states and may also retard aging.

Doctors and chiropractors recommend **strengthening opposing muscle groups**. When we do an action over and over with a particular muscle, that muscle gets very large and strong, creating an imbalance with the muscles surrounding it. This imbalance creates stress and strain. Counterbalancing exercises help in this regard. For example, if you are a pianist, the muscles that make your fingers press the keys downward are likely to be very strong. An opposing exercise might be to forcibly lift the fingers of one hand in an upward motion while using the other hand to provide resistance for those fingers. The concept is to create exercises that are the exact opposite of the actions required when you play.

Surgery should be avoided at all costs. I have <u>never</u> met a musician who underwent surgery for overuse injuries that did not have problems later. Let's take a look at carpal tunnel syndrome for example. Carpal tunnel syndrome is caused from too much congestion inside the carpal tunnel (mostly scar tissue) that impedes nerves and tendons that run through the tunnel. This causes numbness in the fingers. A common surgical treatment is to cut the carpal tunnel open and scrape it clean of scar tissue and other debris.

Think: what happens when you cut or scrape yourself? You develop scar tissue in the area. Carpal tunnel surgery cleans the area free of scar tissue for a while-but only for a little while. The body has been injured by a scalpel and will eventually build-up scar tissue again in the area-perhaps even more than you originally had. Lactic acid crystallizes in injured areas as well. It is <u>not</u> a solution. <u>Don't do it.</u>

Doctors and chiropractors prescribe tennis elbow bands or slings. The recommended time for wearing them vary from doctor to doctor. The idea is to rest an area so it will heal. This is a reasonable theory. My experience is that they cause more problems. Your muscles become weaker and atrophy when they are restricted or immobilized. They can then become re-injured easier when returning to regular chores after weeks of immobilization. Atrophy also causes adhesions in muscle tissue, making them less flexible.

Nonetheless, at some point these items may be suggested to you. I recommend following the doctor's orders and try them for a week or so to see if they help. I have never known a person who swears by them get to a point where they didn't need them anymore.

Topical treatments are good for temporary pain relief but do nothing to solve the actual problem. They are a better choice than anti-inflammatory pills like Advil since there is no danger of ulcers from prolonged use. There are many topical products currently on the market. I have personally used Ben Gay Warming Ice, Ben Gay Pain Relieving Rub, Aspercreme Analgesic Creme Rub, and capsicum patches such as Salonpas-Hot. They provide temporary pain relief by distracting your attention to another area (your skin).

Ultra-sound is often the choice of doctors and chiropractors and theoretically promotes healing through the use of sound waves. The sound waves are directed through the skin by an ultra-sound machine. These sound waves break up scar tissue and adhesions and promote circulation and waste removal. Doctors and chiropractors are the only ones able to purchase the industrial ultra-sound machines. A Japanese consumer ultra-sound device is about $200 to $300. Be sure to avoid using it in an area that doesn't have a lot of muscle between the skin and the bone. The machine can cause pitting of the bone if used too close to it. I haven't found them to be beneficial.

APPENDIX

This appendix lists many popular food and supplements, which vitamins/minerals/properties they are high in, and other benefits obtained from them or special considerations.

Apple cider vinegar: potassium; dissolves calcium in blood.

Apples: vitamin A, vitamin C, bioflavonoids, ellagic acid, fiber (lignans), glutathione, pectin, potassium; quickens digestive elimination, may improve viral immunity, has anti - carcinogenic benefits.

Apricots: vitamin A, vitamin C, fiber, iron, potassium.

Asparagus: vitamin A, vitamin C, enzymes, potassium.

Avocados: vitamin A, vitamin C, pectin, potassium.

Bananas: vitamin A, vitamin B6, vitamin C, fiber, pectin, potassium.

Beets: vitamin A, vitamin C, calcium, carotenes, chlorophyll, vitamin E, potassium; juice the entire beet (especially the stems) for maximum benefit.

Bell/green peppers: bioflavonoids, vitamin C.

Brewer's yeast: Vitamin B6, calcium, chromium, iron.

Broccoli: vitamin A, much of the B complex, bioflavonoids, vitamin C, calcium, enzymes, fiber; has anti - carcinogenic benefits.

Brussels sprouts: vitamin A, vitamin C, calcium, enzymes, fiber, iron, potassium; has anti - carcinogenic benefits.

Cabbage: vitamin A, bioflavonoids, vitamin C, calcium, carotenes (in red cabbage), enzymes, fiber (lignans), potassium; has anti - carcinogenic benefits.

Cantaloupe: vitamin A, bioflavonoids, vitamin C, potassium.

Carrots: vitamin A, vitamin C, calcium, carotenes, vitamin E, enzymes, fiber, glutathione, potassium; improves complexion, cleans waste from the digestive tract, reduces chances of sunburn.

Cauliflower: vitamin A, vitamin C, enzymes, fiber, potassium; has anti - carcinogenic benefits.

Celery: vitamin A, vitamin E, enzymes, fiber, potassium; purifies blood, liver.

Cherries: bioflavonoids, pectin; may help with the prevention of gout.

Corn: vitamin A, potassium, fiber.

Cranberries: bioflavonoids; cleanses blood, kidneys, bladder, fights viruses, and quells inflammation.

Cucumbers: vitamin A, vitamin C, calcium, enzymes, iron, potassium.

Figs: calcium, potassium.

Garlic: vitamin C, calcium.

Grapefruit: vitamin A, bioflavonoids, vitamin C, calcium, fiber, potassium.

Grapes: pectin.

Green beans and peas: vitamin A, much of the B complex, vitamin C, calcium, enzymes, fiber, iron, magnesium, potassium, protein, zinc.

Guavas: vitamin C.

Kale: vitamin A, much of the B complex, vitamin C, calcium, carotenes, chlorophyll, enzymes, fiber, potassium.

Lecithin: phosphatides; purifies bloodstream, may help memory, dissolves lactic acid.

Lemons: bioflavonoids, vitamin C, potassium; an anonic food.

Lettuce: vitamin A, vitamin C, calcium, chlorophyll, enzymes, potassium; has anti - carcinogenic benefits.

Limes: bioflavonoids, vitamin C.

Mushrooms: enzymes.

Oatmeal: fiber.

Onions: vitamin A, bioflavonoids, vitamin C, calcium, potassium, prostaglandin.

Oranges: vitamin A, bioflavonoids, vitamin C, calcium, potassium.

Papayas: bioflavonoids, vitamin C, fiber; speeds cellular production.

Parsley: vitamin A, much of the B complex, vitamin C, calcium, carotenes, chlorophyll, enzymes, iron, potassium; has anti - carcinogenic benefits.

Peaches: vitamin A, bioflavonoids, vitamin C, fiber, pectin, potassium.

Peanuts: vitamin B6.

Pears: fiber, potassium.

Pineapples: vitamin A, vitamin C, fiber, pectin; dissolves mucus.

Plums: bioflavonoids, carotenes.

Potatoes: vitamin A, bioflavonoids, vitamin C, carotenes, fiber, iron, potassium; eat the skin, too.

Prunes: vitamin A, fiber, potassium.

Raisins: iron, fiber, pectin.

Raspberries: bioflavonoids, pectin; cleanses bloodstream.

Sesame seeds: iron, pectin.

Spinach: vitamin A, much of the B complex, vitamin C, calcium, carotenes, chlorophyll, fiber, glutathione, iron, octacosanol.

Squash: vitamin A, vitamin C, calcium, enzymes, fiber, iron, potassium.

Strawberries: bioflavonoids, vitamin C, ellagic acid, cleans the bloodstream, has anti - carcinogenic benefits.

Sunflower seeds: calcium, iron, pectin.

Tangerines: vitamin A, bioflavonoids, vitamin C, calcium, potassium.

Tomatoes: vitamin A, vitamin B6, bioflavonoids, vitamin C, carotenes, enzymes, fiber, pectin, potassium.

Turnips: vitamin C, calcium, enzymes, fiber, potassium; has anti - carcinogenic benefits; be sure to juice the entire turnip (including leaves).

Wheat germ: vitamin B6, fiber (lignans), octacosanol; speeds waste elimination and body repair times.

Yams: calcium, fiber, iron, potassium.

BIBLIOGRAPHY

Robert A. and Jean E. Anderson. *Stretching.*
Shelter Publications, Inc.,
Bolinas, California; 1980.

Cherie Calbom/Maureen Keane. *Juicing For Life.*
Avery Publishing Group,
New York; 1992.

Annemarie Colbin. *Food and Healing.*
Ballantine Books,
New York; 1986.

William Dufty. *Sugar Blues.*
Warner Books,
New York; 1975.

Bonnie Prudden. *Pain Erasure: The Bonnie Prudden Way.*
Ballantine Books,
New York; 1980.

William Schultz. *Japanese Finger Pressure Therapy: Do It Yourself Accupressure.*
Bell Publishing Company,
New York.

Carlson Wade. *Inner Cleansing.*
Parker Publishing Company,
New York; 1983.

Julie Lyonn Lieberman, W. Donald Cooke. *You Are Your Instrument: The Definitive Musician's Guide to Practice and Performance.*
Music Sales Corporation,
New York; 1992.

About the Author:

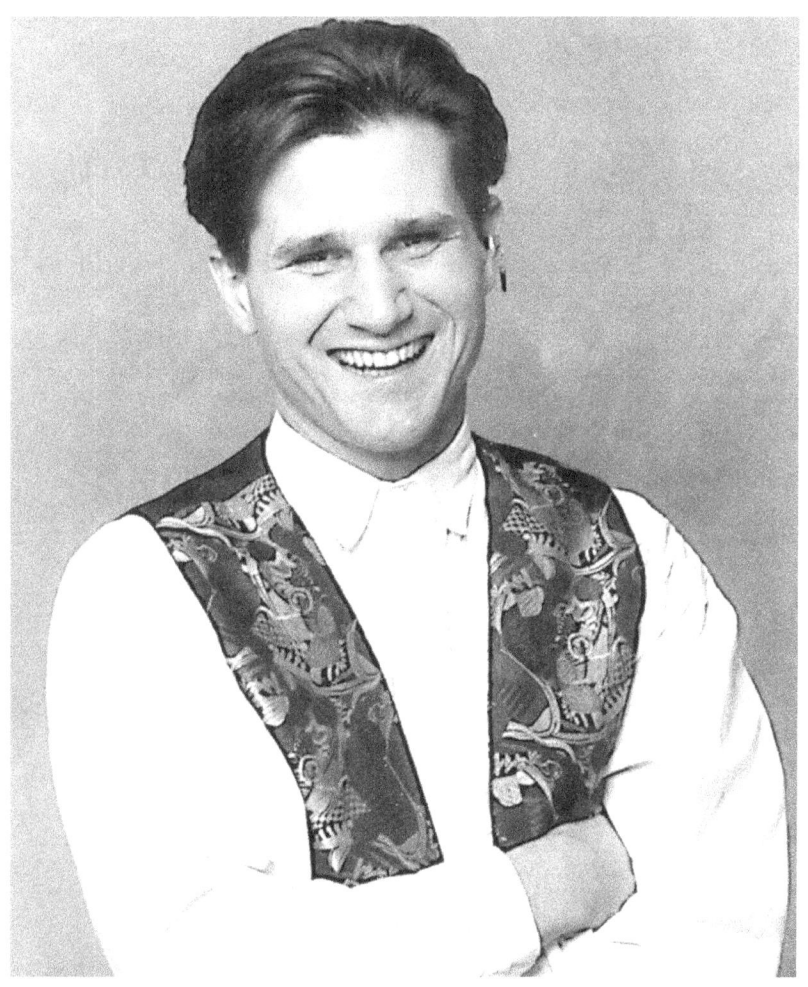

David Enos has established himself as one of Los Angeles' top bassists. His talents have been honed through extensive work with artists like Arturo Sandoval, Sergio Mendes, David Benoit, Bobby Caldwell, Frank Gambale, Nelson Rangel, Danilo Perez, Stan Getz, Alphonse Mouzon, and a host of others. In addition, his basswork has been heard on Chevrolet and Honda commercials, Charlie Brown television specials, BET (Black Entertainment Television), and many other shows. David had an eight - year bout with tendonitis, carpal tunnel syndrome, and bone spurs after an excessive six month practice regimen. This eight - year period found him going to various health specialists for help: everyone from doctors to chiropractors to myotherapy to acupuncture. Although told repeatedly that chronic overuse injuries are permanent, David never stopped searching for answers to his problems. Eventually his perseverance paid off through combining the most effective advice he could from various health fields. David currently lives completely pain - free in the Los Angeles area with his wife and three children. The book you hold in your hands is a culmination of his eight - year ordeal with overuse injuries.

David Enos exclusively uses BSX electric upright basses, Bossa electric basses, Polytone amplifiers, Slider Dual Shoulder straps, and Labella strings.